This book has been sponsored by Ethicon Endo-Surgery (Europe) GmbH and Johnson & Johnson MEDICAL GmbH, Norderstedt, Germany. The authors are responsible for the content of the publication. Information provided in this book is offered in good faith as an educational tool for health care professionals. The information has been thoroughly reviewed and is believed to be useful and accurate at the time of its publication, but is offered without warranty of any kind. The authors and the sponsors shall not be responsible for any loss or damage arising from its use. Always refer to the instructions for use that comes with each device for the most current and complete instructions.

OPERATION PRIMER volume 11

Laparoscopic Sleeve Gastrectomy

Editors

Marc Immenroth
Jürgen Brenner

Authors

Rudolf A. Weiner
Ralph Peterli

assisted by

Indre Offermann

Maike Aukstinnis
Ann-Katrin Güler
Astrid Künemund
Annegret Röhling
Detlev Ruge

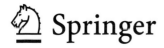
Springer

Authors

Rudolf A. Weiner, M.D.
Head of Surgical Department, Krankenhaus Frankfurt Sachsenhausen,
EU-IFSO certificated Center for Surgery of Obesity and Metabolic Disorders,
Schulstr. 31,
60594 Frankfurt a.M., Germany

Ralph Peterli, M.D.
Associate Professor of Surgery, St. Claraspital AG,
Kleinriehenstrasse 30,
4058 Basel, Switzerland

Editors

Marc Immenroth, PhD
Senior Marketing Manager EP Germany & Plus Platform & Synthetic Absorbables D-A-CH,
Johnson & Johnson MEDICAL GmbH,
Robert-Koch-Straße 1,
22851 Norderstedt, Germany

Jürgen Brenner, MD
Managing Director
Eric Krauthammer & Dr. Jürgen Brenner
Creative Team-Leadership

ISBN 978-3-642-23889-5 Laparoscopic Sleeve Gastrectomy

Bibliografische Information der Deutschen Bibliothek
The Deutsche Bibliothek lists this publication in Deutsche Nationalbibliographie;
detailed bibliographic data are available in the internet at http://dnb.ddb.de.

First published in Germany in 2012 by Springer Medizin Verlag
springer.com

© Ethicon Endo-Surgery (Europe) GmbH

SPIN 80112611
Layout and typesetting: Dr. Carl GmbH, Stuttgart, Germany
Printing: Stürtz GmbH, Würzburg, Germany

18/5135/DK – 5 4 3 2 1 0

EDITORS' PREFACE

This Operation Primer marks the continuation of a series of very successful books, which have gained ever more recognition in recent years. Thanks to consistently positive reviews in renowned specialist publications in both England and Germany, we are motivated to continue to invest in these 'cook books' for surgeons. In response to international demand we plan to release the forthcoming English-language primers in other languages. In addition to the central European languages. Chinese will also be available.

The idea for the Operation Primer series originated in a scientific study entitled "Mental Training in Surgical Education" that formed part of a collaborative project between the surgical department of the University of Cologne, the Institute of Sports and Sports Science of the University of Heidelberg and the European Surgical Institute (ESI) in Norderstedt. The aim of the study was to evaluate the effect of mental training, which has been used successfully in top-class sports for decades, on surgical training. However, in order for mental training to be applied to surgery, it first had to undergo modification. In the course of this modification, the first Operation Primer was produced, the layout of which was largely adopted for the final version presented here. The practice of defining nodal points for operations and then learning these by heart and going through them mentally has been proven to lead to better surgical results. Surgeons approach operations more prepared, are no longer surprised when confronted with the unexpected, and thus operate with more confidence.

We are pleased to complete the "Trilogy" of bariatric surgery Operation Primers with this issue focusing on sleeve gastrectomy. Morbid obesity is a problem and is becoming more and more important. The high number of affected patients with extensive co-morbidities has assumed pandemic proportions.

The operative therapy after exhaustion of more conservative methods is recognized as a safe and effective treatment. The minimally invasive approach has greatly minimized the risk of infection and incisional hernias. Like other minimally invasive procedures, the gastric sleeve procedure is technically complex with a corresponding learning curve.

This Operation Primer should help you, step-by-step, nodal point for nodal point, to increase the safety of the surgical intervention. We have had the pleasure of working with *Rudolf Weiner* and *Ralph Peterli,* two renowned and highly skilled experts, as authors. We are especially pleased that *Henry Buchwald,* the father of bariatric surgery, has honored this book with a foreword.

We have also received excellent support from *Dr. Carl GmbH,* which has accompanied us at each stage of the working process and has contributed greatly to making these innovative surgical textbooks what they are. The diagrams, line drawings, etc. were produced mainly by *Thomas Heller.* *Detlev Ruge* was responsible for the pictures featured in this Operation Primer. The existing concept of practical surgical primers has become reality through the publishing company *Springer Medizin Verlag Heidelberg.* Sincere thanks to all of them.

Practical training is an indispensable prerequisite of safe operating, much in line with this thought from Confucius:

"Tell me, I'll forget; Show me, I may remember; Involve me, I'll understand."

The Editors   January 2012

AUTHORS' PREFACE

This operation primer marks the continuation of a series of successful books, which cover various fields of surgery, including obesity and metabolic disorders. After publishing guidebooks for laparoscopic adjustable gastric banding and gastric bypass, we are pleased to offer the latest addition focusing on sleeve gastrectomy.

Worldwide, sleeve gastrectomy is becoming an increasingly popular procedure in the treatment of obesity. Initially introduced as a component of complex interventions, such as the biliopancreatic diversion with duodenal switch (DS), and later as part of a two-stage operation in high-risk patients, the procedure is now more common as a one-stage operation and the subject of avid scientific discussion.

The concept of longitudinal gastric resection is not new. The procedure was first established in ulcer surgery in the 1920's and reintroduced in the 1960's by M. Saegesser, a fellow of Ernst Heller, but thereafter faded in popularity. The modern procedure of longitudinal gastric resection, also known as sleeve gastrectomy, was incorporated quite late into the repertoire of obesity surgery. In 1993, P. Marceau and co-workers modified biliopancreatic diversion, originally introduced by N. Scopinaro. They replaced horizontal gastric resection with longitudinal gastric resection on the side of greater curvature, combining preservation of the pylorus and doubling the length of the "common tract" to 100 cm.

The first laparoscopic BPD-DS was performed in 1999 by M. Gagner along with the first laparoscopic sleeve gastrectomy (LSG). Frequent complications and a high mortality rate in patients with a high BMI (> 60 kg/m^2) led to a two-step procedure: first, LSG and after significant weight loss, the second step was performed under better conditions with increased safety for the patient. However, due to sufficient weight loss and high patient satisfaction, a number of patients did not reappear for the second procedure.

These experiences in the United States, Belgium and Germany were the basis for introduction of the LSG as a single-stage procedure into the spectrum of procedures in the treatment of morbid obesity. The value of sleeve gastrectomy within the spectrum of surgical weight loss and metabolic procedures is still under discussion. While not the preferred universal procedure for bariatric surgery, experience and success from other procedures simplified and facilitated the development of sleeve gastrectomy, offering a potentially attractive treatment option.

The apparent simplicity of the sleeve gastrectomy procedure is deceptive. This operation primer will provide you with detailed descriptions of the current technique and important steps to prevent complications. Although obesity surgery has proven to be the most effective treatment for morbid obesity, surgical techniques are not infallible. In an effort to improve reliability, several surgeons started to change the techniques used. The actual consensus in performing LSG is documented in this operation primer.

Rudolf A. Weiner
Ralph Peterli

January 2012

"Intellectual expertise can be proven with papers,
but one can only trust someone who speaks from experience."

Hermann Hesse (1877–1962), German poet, 1946 Nobel Prize for Literature

… with this in mind, the editors are especially pleased that Henry Buchwald
agreed to write the guest foreword for this book.

Gastric plication, described by Tretbar in 1976, and gastric wrapping, described by Wilkinson and Pelosi in 1981, were the predecessors of the sleeve gastrectomy, which was described by Marceau et al. in 1993, and Hess in 1998, as part of their adaptation of Scopinaro's biliopancreatic diversion (BPD) to a duodenal switch (DS). De Csepel et al succeeded in performing BPD/DS laparoscopically in a porcine model in 2001, but, when attempting the procedure clinically experienced a high complication rate, causing them to advocate a two-stage procedure with the sleeve gastrectomy as the initial stage. Though open, laparoscopic, and even robotic BPD/DS have now been mastered with minimal complications, serendipitously it was recognized that after the first-stage sleeve gastrectomy certain patients manifested good weight loss at one year, causing indefinite postponement, and subsequent abandonment, of the second stage of the BPD/DS. Since 2003, laparoscopic sleeve gastrectomy as a stand-alone operation has found many advocates. By 2008, over 5% of bariatric procedures worldwide were sleeve gastrectomies, and that number is increasing rapidly.

With the appreciation that bariatric surgery is metabolic surgery, came recognition that resection of the greater gastric curvature is more than anatomically and functionally restrictive. This resection alters the hormonal milieu of the intestinal tract, in particular decreasing ghrelin secretion, as well as removing the normal gastric pacemaker and influencing the nerve syncytium of the foregut. What effects these changes have on hunger, satiety, and type 2 diabetes are, as yet, poorly understood.

The technique of sleeve gastrectomy is to establish a tubular gastric conduit from the esophagus to the pylorus by dividing the short gastric vessels and resecting the greater curvature aspect of the stomach with an intra-luminal bougie as a guide. Certain surgeons start the dissection opposite the pes anserinus; others start at the pylorus; the resection is ended short of the esophagogastric junction. The gastric staple line can be reinforced with hemostatic strips of various compositions, or by oversewing.

The acute hazards of sleeve gastrectomy per se are primarily that of a staple line leak, followed by staple line bleeding and constriction of the retained gastric conduit. Due to removal of the gastric pacemaker, patients may experience distress on eating, inability to propel food beyond their gastric tube, and vomiting for several weeks, all without any evidence of obstruction.

Early and medium-term follow-up of sleeve gastrectomy series indicates a mean excess weight loss and resolution of comorbidities (type 2 diabetes, hyperlipidemia, hypertension) somewhere between laparoscopic adjustable gastric banding and gastric bypass. There are, as yet, few studies with a follow-up greater than 5 years. Ultimate evaluation and judgment of sleeve gastrectomy outcomes will need to wait for long-term data to become available.

In the event that weight is regained, it is not difficult to revise a sleeve revision to a gastric bypass, or to perform a completion operation to a DS. It is prudent and ethical to warn sleeve gastrectomy patients prior to surgery that it may become necessary for them to undergo a second procedure in order to maintain or to achieve adequate weight loss.

The Primer Series, edited by Marc Immenroth and Jürgen Brenner, deserve recognition and credit for teaching tools providing step-by-step illustrated guidance. This particular Operation Primer on sleeve gastrectomy should be read by all surgeons contemplating or actually engaged in performing sleeve gastrectomies.

There can be no better authors for this succinct and definitive exposition of sleeve gastrectomy than Rudolf Weiner and Ralph Peterli. Both are technically highly skilled surgeons with years of experience in performing metabolic/bariatric surgery. They are students and teachers of metabolic/bariatric surgery, with multiple and significant literature contributions. Their opinions and contributions are globally respected.

Henry Buchwald
University of Minnesota   January 2012

Rudolf A. Weiner, M.D.

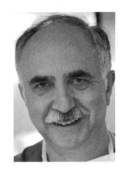

- Studied medicine at the University of Leipzig, Germany
- 1976 Doctorate in medicine at the University of Leipzig, Germany
- 1977–1984 Training in general surgery at the Hospital of „St.Georg" Leipzig, Germany
- 1981 Research doctorate at the University of Berlin, Germany
- 1981 Qualified as a urologist
- 1984 Qualified as a general surgeon
- 1993–2000 Senior surgeon at the Hospital Nordwest, Frankfurt am Main, Germany
- 2000 Professor of surgery at Johann Wolfgang Goethe-University, Frankfurt am Main, Germany
- 2001 Director of the Department of Surgery at the Frankfurt Sachsenhausen Hospital and Center for Minimally Invasive Surgery, Germany
- 2010–2012 President of the European Chapter of IFSO
- 2011 President of the World Congress of IFSO

Focus of Research and Work
- Received specific obesity surgery training
- Performed advanced laparoscopic surgery as early as June 1990
- First laparoscopic gastric banding 1994
- Developed and standardized the surgical technique for the laparoscopic application of gastric banding (LAP-BAND) „Pars flaccida technique"
- Regularly performs live procedures in front of audiences worldwide
- Teaches at Johann Wolfgang Goethe-University, Frankfurt am Main
- Organized regular international workshops where over 750 surgeons worldwide were given hands-on training on the laparoscopic obesity and metabolic surgery
- President of the Live-Surgery-Meeting (Frankfurt Meeting for surgery of obesity and metabolic disorders) since 1998
- Performs all bariatric procedures (more than 4500 cases since 1993)
- Principal investigator in the project TANTALUS (gastric stimulation) and telemetric gastric banding (Easy-Band)

Memberships
- Society of American Gastrointestinal Endoscopic Surgeons (SAGES)
- International Federation of Surgery for Obesity and Metabolic Disoders (IFSO) – Executive Council (2010–2012), President of EU-Chapter (2010–2012)
- European Association for Endoscopic Surgery (EAES)
- American Society for Bariatric Surgery and Metabolic Disorders (ASMBS)
- German Society for Surgery
- German Society for Bariatric Surgery (President, 2006)
- Editorial Boards: Bariatric Times, Adipositas (Schattauer), Chirurgische Allgemeine
- Co-Editor: Obesity Surgery, Obesity Facts, Adipositasspektrum
- Chairman of the Consortium for Obesity Therapy (2007–2010, 2010–2013)
- Member of the German Society for General and Visceral Surgery Committee (2007–2010, 2010–2013)
- German Society for Obesity, Advisory Board (2008–present)

Author and Co-Author of many scientific articles in journals around the world including Surgical Endoscopy, Obesity Surgery, Surgical Laparoscopy & Endoscopy, International Surgery, Hepato-Gastroenterology, Der Chirurg, Chirurgische Allgemeine and other

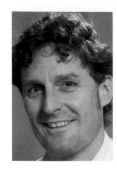

Ralph Peterli, M.D.

- Studied medicine at the University of Basel, Switzerland
- 1988 Doctorate in medicine at the University of Basel, Switzerland
- 1995 Qualified as a general surgeon
- 2004 Subspecialized in General and Trauma Surgery
- 2004 Subspecialized in Visceral Surgery
- 2009 Assistant Professor of Surgery, University of Basel, Switzerland

Focus of Research and Work
- Teacher at the Medical School of the University of Basel
- Metabolic surgery
- Various clinical studies in bariatric surgery
- Various clinical studies on laparoscopic cholecystectomy and related hepato-biliary pathologies
- Main investigator of a multi-centre prospective randomized trial comparing laparoscopic sleeve gastrectomy with laparaoscopic Roux-en-Y gastric bypass
- Adipokines in morbidly obese patients undergoing bariatric surgery
- Glycemic control and gastrointestinal peptides in morbidly obese patients
- Proteomics of mitochondria in human adipose tissue
- Human adipose tissue and functional role of melanocortin-receptors
- 3 national and 1 international scientific prizes

Memberships
- Swiss Study Group for Morbid Obesity (SMOB), board member, treasurer
- International Federation of Surgery of Obesity (IFSO), European council member
- Consensus Adipositas Schweiz, editorial member
- Editorial board: Obesity Surgery
- Swiss medical Society (FMH)
- Swiss Surgical Society (SGC)
- Medical Society Basel (MEDGES)
- American Society of Bariatric Surgery (ASMBS)
- Société internationale de chirurgie (SIC)
- Breast Surgery Society (BSI/Senologie)
- Schweizerische Arbeitsgemeinschaft für laparoskopische und thorakoskopische Chirurgie (SALTC)
- Schweizerische Gesellschaft für Allgemeine Chirurgie und Unfallchirurgie (SGAUC)

Author and Co-Author of many scientific articles, book chapters, abstracts and invited lectures

Contents

Appendices

Introduction

From an educational point of view, the Operation Primer is somewhat plagiaristic. The layout – and this can be admitted freely – is taken over largely from commonly available cook books. In such books, the ingredients and cooking utensils required to prepare the recipe in question are normally listed first. The most important cooking procedures are then described briefly in the text. Photographs support the written explanations and show what the dish should look like when prepared. Sometimes diagrams and illustrations make individual cooking steps clearer.

Despite these obvious parallels, there is a crucial difference between cook books and the Operation Primer: in the Operation Primer, complicated and complex surgical techniques are described that are intended to help the surgeon and his team perform an operation safely and economically. Ultimately, it always comes down to the patient's welfare. The following must therefore be said early in this introduction:

- The use of the Operation Primer as an aid to operating requires that surgical techniques have first been completely mastered.

- Being alert to possible mistakes is categorically the most important principle when operating; avoiding mistakes is crucial.

As already mentioned in the Editors' preface, the concept of the Operation Primer originated in a scientific study with the title "Mental Training in Surgical Education" that formed part of a collaborative project between the surgical department of the University of Cologne (under Prof. Hans Troidl), the Institute of Sports and Sports Science of the University of Heidelberg, and the European Surgical Institute (ESI) in Norderstedt. Laparoscopic cholecystectomy was the initial focus.

Mental training is derived from top-class sports. This is understood as methodically repeating and consciously imagining actions and movements without actually carrying them out at the same time (cf. Driskell, Copper & Moran, 1994; Feltz & Landers, 1983; Immenroth, 2003; Immenroth, Eberspächer & Hermann, 2008). Scientific involvement with imagining movement has a long tradition in medical and psychological research. As early as 1852, Lotze described how imagining and perceiving movements can lead to a concurrent performance "with quiet movements …" (Lotze, 1852). This phenomenon later became known by the names "Ideomotion" and "Carpenter effect" (Carpenter, 1874).

In the collaborative project, mental training was modified in such a way that it could be employed in the training and further education of young surgeons. In mental training in surgery, surgeons visualize the operation from the inner perspective without performing any actual movements, i.e., they go through the operation step by step in their mind's eye. In the study that was conducted at the ESI, the first Operation Primer was used as the basis for this visualization. In this primer, laparoscopic cholecystectomy was subdivided into individual, clearly depicted steps, the so-called nodal points.

The study evaluated the effect of the mental training on learning laparoscopic cholecystectomy compared with practical training and with a control group. The planning, conduct, and evaluation of the study took 7 years (2000–2007), with over 100 surgeons participating.

The results corresponded exactly with the expectations: the mentally trained surgeons improved in a similar degree to those surgeons who received additional practical training on a pelvi trainer simulator (in some subscales even more). Moreover, there was greater improvement in these two groups compared with the control group, which did not receive any additional mental or practical training (cf. in detail, Immenroth, Bürger, Brenner, Nagelschmidt, Eberspächer & Troidl, 2007;

Immenroth, Bürger, Brenner, Kemmler, Nagelschmidt, Eberspächer & Troidl, 2005; Immenroth, Eberspächer, Nagelschmidt, Troidl, Bürger, Brenner, Berg, Müller & Kemmler, 2005).

Recently, a significant improvement in surgical knowledge and confidence was shown by both experienced and novice surgeons in another study about mental training in laparoscopic surgery (Arora et al., 2010). Therefore, mental training can be seen as a cost- and time-effective training tool that should be integrated into surgical training.

Furthermore, the study by Immenroth et al. (2007) included a questionnaire to determine the extent to which the mentally trained surgeons accepted mental training as a teaching method in surgery. Mental training was assessed as very positive by all 34 mentally trained surgeons. The Operation Primer received particular acclaim in the evaluation:

- 82 % of the surgeons wished to use similar self-made Operation Primers in their daily work.

- 85 % of the surgeons attributed the success of the mental training at least in part to the Operation Primer.

- 88 % of the surgeons wanted to have these Operation Primers as a fixed component of the course at the ESI.

This positive response to the study was the starting point for the production of the present series of Operation Primers.

Prior to publication, the Operation Primer was developed by methodical and didactical means and then adapted to the readers' needs and wishes. This was carried out following a survey of 93 surgeons (interns, resident doctors, assistant medical directors and medical directors) who participated in surgical courses at the ESI. They evaluated in detail the structure and components by means of a questionnaire.

The results of this survey gave important findings on how to optimize the Operation Primer. The sense and representation of the nodal points, the comprehensibility and detail of the text, and the photographs of the operation were highly valued especially by young surgeons (Güler, Immenroth, Berg, Bürger & Gawad, 2006). The comprehensive research undertaken with this Operation Primer series will ensure its overall value to the reader.

Structure and handling of the Operation Primer

In the present series of Operation Primers, an attempt has been made to standardize the described laparoscopic operations as much as possible. This is achieved first by applying the same format to all operating techniques described. Second, operative sequences that are performed identically in all operations are always explained using the same blocks of text. By following a general structure for the description of all operations and by using identical text blocks, it was intended to aid recognition of recurring patterns and their translation into action even for different operations.

The Operation Primer is divided into five chapters, each identified by Roman numerals and different register colors in the margin. The contents of the individual chapters will now be explained.

In **Preparations for the operation**, the basic instruments for all laparoscopic operations and then the additional instruments for the specific operation are listed. This is followed by a detailed description of the positioning and shaving of the patient, attaching the dispersive electrode, setting up the equipment, skin disinfection and sterile draping of the patient. The operative preparation is concluded with a detailed description and an illustration of how the operating team is to be positioned for the operation in question.

In the chapter **Creating the pneumoperitoneum – placing the trocar for the scope**, three alternatives are shown in detail: the Hasson method, trocar with optical obturator, and Veress needle. The choice of method is up to the individual surgeon. All three alternatives are employed in surgical practice. However, it should be pointed out that the greatest danger in minimally invasive surgery is the insertion of the Veress needle, as it is done "blind".

3 possibilities for creating the pneumoperitoneum: the choice is up to the surgeon

Veress needle = greatest danger!

Placing the working trocars is explained in detail in the next chapter. The written explanations are supplemented by a diagram. In order to keep a constant overview of the placement of the trocars, even during the following description of the operation sequence, this illustration is shown in diminished size in every single operative step.

Continuous illustration of the trocar positions

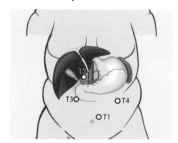

The core of the Operation Primer is the chapter **Nodal points**. This is where the actual sequence of the operation is described in detail. However, prior to this detailed explanation, the term nodal point will be explained briefly. In the Editors' preface and introduction, mental training was mentioned as a form of training used successfully in top-class sports for decades, and this is where the term originates. In sports as in surgery, a nodal point is understood as one of those structural components of movement that are absolutely essential for performing the movement optimally. Nodal points have to be passed through in succession and are characterized by a reduction in the degrees of freedom of action. In mental training they act as orientation points for methodical repetition and conscious imagining of the athletic or operative movement (cf. in detail Immenroth et al., 2008).

Nodal point = term from top-class sports

Nodal points:
1) absolutely essential
2) successive order
3) no degrees of freedom

For every operation in the Operation Primer series, these nodal points were extracted in a prolonged process by the authors in collaboration with the editors. The nodal points represent the basic structural framework of an operation. Because of their particular relevance and for better orientation, all of the nodal points in the Operation Primer are shown on the left on each double page as a flow chart. The current nodal point is highlighted graphically. The instruments required for this nodal point and the specific trocars for it are listed in a box on the right, beside the flow chart.

Flow chart of the sequence of nodal points on each double page

Below the instrument box, instructions regarding the nodal point are given as briefly as possible. According to Miller (1956), people can best store 7±2 units of information ("Magical number 7"). Therefore, no more than seven single instructions are listed per nodal point, if possible. With re-

Maximum of 7±2 instructions per nodal point

gard to the instructions, it should be noted that the change of instruments between the individual nodal points is not described explicitly as a rule; rather, this is apparent through different instruments in the instrument box.

Watch-outs are pointed out in red!

Where necessary, particular moments where special attention is needed are pointed out in red.

Alternatives: In small blue print at the end of the nodal point.

The described operation sequence is only one way of performing the operation safely and economically, namely the way preferred by the authors. Undoubtedly, a number of other equally valid operation sequences exist. As far as possible, notes on alternative methods are given in small blue print at the end of each nodal point.

In the fifth chapter, the **Management of difficult situations and complications** is described in detail. In general, details on adhesions, bleeding, injuries to organs, etc. are given first.

Illustration of anatomical variations, an example of an operation note, postoperative management, and postoperative complications in the appendices

In the **Appendices** relevant anatomical variations which can occur in the operation sequence and may require a different approach are described first. In order to give the Operation Primer even more practical relevance, an example of an operation note is then reproduced. The appendices also contain helpful hints for using a circular stapler as a variation of the gastric bypass procedure, detailed information about the postoperative management, postoperative complications and their management, as well as the bibliographical references and list of keywords.

(→ p. 60, V-4) = reference to the 4th section of chapter V

In order to avoid repetition, reference is made throughout the text to relevant chapters of the Operation Primer, if necessary. To do this, the Roman numeral of the chapter and the number of the corresponding section are shown in parentheses. Referral is made most often to the fifth chapter, where the management of difficult situations and complications is described. These references are set off in red letters.

All sources in the literature are listed in the bibliography

Finally, it must be pointed out that for better readability of the Operation Primer no bibliographical references at all are given in the text. However, in order to give an overview of the basic and more extensive sources, the entire literature is listed in the bibliography.

Make sure that the following preoperative requirements for laparoscopic sleeve gastrectomy have been met:

- The indication for the operation is correct.

- The patient has given detailed informed written consent.

- The bowel is prepared appropriately prior to laparoscopic gastrointestinal surgery.

- Thromboprophylaxis (low-molecular-weight heparin, compression stockings) has been given as per local practice.

- Single-dose perioperative antibiotic prophylaxis has been given.

Basic instruments

- Size 11 scalpel
- 10 ml syringe with 0.9 % NaCl solution
- Dissecting scissors
- 2 Langenbeck hooks
- Suction device
- Needle holder
- Suture scissors
- 2 surgical forceps
- 2 Backhaus clamps
- Compresses
- Swabs with an integral X-ray contrast strip
- Sutures:
    - Fascia: 2–0 absorbable, polyfilament, if necessary
    - Subcutaneous: 3–0 absorbable, polyfilament, if necessary
    - Skin: 4–0 or 5–0 absorbable, monofilament or a skin stapler
- Trocar side closure device, if necessary
- Skin adhesive, if necessary
- Dressings

Instruments for the first access, depending on the type of access:

a) Hasson method:
    - Hasson trocar (10/12 mm)
    - 2 retaining sutures (2–0)
    - Purse-string suture (2–0)

b) Trocar with optical obturator (e.g. Endopath XCEL® bladeless trocar, Ethicon Endo-Surgery)

c) Veress needle (e.g. Endopath® Ultra Veress Insufflation Needle, Ethicon Endo-Surgery)

> **There should always be a basic laparotomy set in the operating room so that in an emergency a laparotomy can be performed without delay!**

Additional instruments for laparoscopic sleeve gastrectomy

Trocars: (e.g. Endopath XCEL® trocar, Ethicon Endo-Surgery)
T1: Trocar for the scope   (10/12 mm)
T2: Working trocar   (5 mm or 10/12 mm; depending on the liver retracting device)
T3: Working trocar   (10/12 mm)
T4: Working trocar   (10/12 mm)

- Additional trocars, if necessary
- Reducer caps, if necessary
- Angled scope 30° (0° scope, if necessary, for trocar with optical obturator)

Extra-long trocars should always be available.

- 2 atraumatic grasping forceps (10 mm)
- Ultrasonic dissector (e.g. Harmonic® shears, Ethicon Endo-Surgery)
- Extra-long HF (high-frequency) electrode handle and hook
- Endoscopic linear cutter (e.g. Echelon Flex™ Endopath® Stapler, articulating endoscopic linear cutter 45 mm, Ethicon Endo-Surgery)
- Different cartridges (depending on tissue thickness)
- Liver retracting device with fixation arm
- Additional liver retracting device with fixation arm, if necessary
- Curved dissector
- Dissecting swab
- Curved scissors
- Needle holder
- Sutures: 1–0 absorbable, polyfilament
- Suction-irrigation instrument
- Retrieval pouch (e.g. Endopouch Retriever®, Ethicon Endo-Surgery)

For the anesthetist:
- Gastric calibration tube 180° asymmetrical balloon (e.g. Gastric Calibration Tube Obtech, Ethicon Endo-Surgery*)
- 5 ml methylene blue 1 %
- 10 ml syringe with cannula
- Small bowl

Please always refer to the instructions for use that comes with each device for the most current and complete instructions.

*Manufactured by Obtech Medical Sàrl and marketed by Ethicon Endo-Surgery

Basic instruments

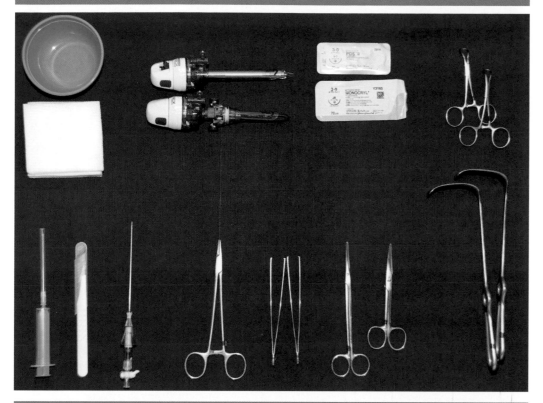

Additional instruments for laparoscopic sleeve gastrectomy

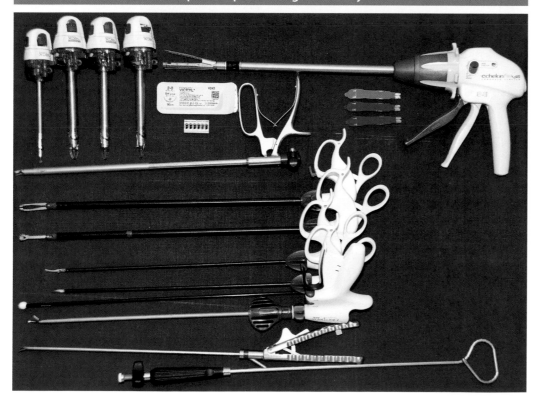

Emptying the urinary bladder

- In order to achieve excellent exposure of the small pelvis and to avoid injuries to the urinary bladder, make sure that the patient's bladder is emptied preoperatively by placing a temporary transurethral catheter.

Positioning of the patient

The technical fittings, especially the operating table, must be approved and functional for the patient's weight!

- Position the patient in the lithotomy position.

- Stretch thighs and legs apart with a slight flexure.

- Place both arms at an angle no greater than 70° to the long axis of the body in order to avoid injuries to the axillary nerves.

- Pad the shoulders, elbows and knee joints in order to avoid pressure injuries, particularly of the nerves.

- For better positioning of the patient, hyperextend the back in the lumbar region with a pad. Adjust the operating table appropriately.

- Use a padded board as a surface to lie on to prevent the patient from sliding when put in extreme positions.

- The appropriate positioning should be tested before the sterile draping is performed.

- After creating the pneumoperitoneum and inserting the trocar for the scope (→ p. 25, II) and the scope (→ p. 30, III), position the patient in a reverse Trendelenburg position (30°–45°).

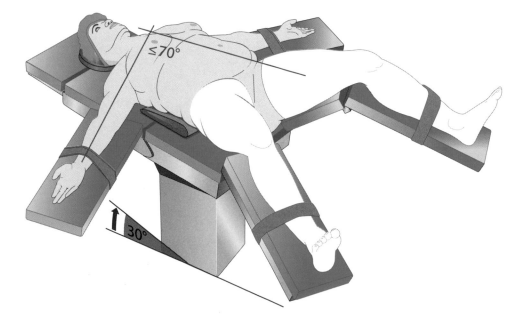

Shaving

- Shave the patient from the mamillae to above the pubic symphysis and from the left to the right anterior superior iliac spine in order to be able to convert to a conventional operation if complications occur.

- If monopolar current is used, shave the application site of the dispersive electrode (as close as possible to the operating field, e.g. on the upper thigh).

Alternative: Instead of shaving, the hair can be removed by cutting off with scissors or with depilatory cream.

Dispersive electrode

- Before placing the dispersive electrode, ensure that the skin at this site and all skin areas in contact with the table are absolutely dry.

- Then stick the entire surface of the electrode carefully above the greatest possible muscle mass (e.g. on the upper thigh). The conducting cable must be at the greatest possible distance from the operating field.

When using monopolar current, always guard against burns on moist areas of the skin due to current!

Setting up the equipment

- Set the generators of the Harmonic® shears and of the HF electrode to an appropriate power level for the intended use.

- Position the foot pedals, if used.

- Attach the suction-irrigation instrument.

- Select a maximum pressure of 15 mmHg on the CO_2 insufflator (with a flow of more than 20 l/min). There are special insufflators for surgery in extreme obesity with a maximum of 45 l/min available. If this special insufflator is not available, two insufflators can be used.

Generator GEN11 for Harmonic® shears (Ethicon Endo-Surgery)

Skin disinfection

- Disinfect the skin from the mamillae to the pubic symphysis. Pay particular attention to careful disinfection of all skin folds.

Sterile draping

- Drape the operating field with sterile drapes so that it is limited cranially at the level of the xiphoid, just above the umbilicus caudally, and by the midaxillary lines laterally.

- During sterile draping of the operating field, position the fixation arm of the liver retracting device at the right side of the table at the level of the liver.

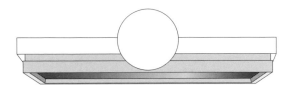

Positioning of the operating team

- The surgeon stands or sits between the patient's spread legs.

- The camera assistant stands to the left at the level of the patient's pelvis.

- The scrub nurse stands to the right, at the level of the patient's knee.

- The monitor is located in the line of vision of the surgeon and the camera assistant on the right at the level of the patient's head.

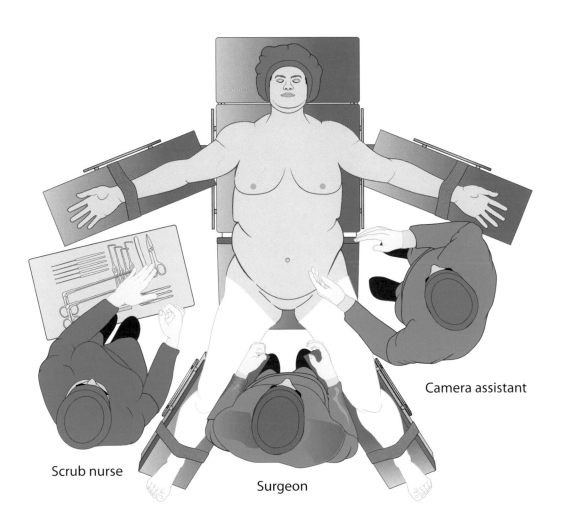

Camera assistant

Scrub nurse

Surgeon

Alternative: If a ceiling monitor is not available, position the monitor in the line of vision of the surgeon and the camera assistant on the right at the level of the patient's head.

CREATING THE PNEUMOPERITONEUM – PLACING THE TROCAR FOR THE SCOPE

Creating the pneumoperitoneum – placing the trocar for the scope

There are three ways of creating a pneumoperitoneum, which will be described in detail below:

a) Hasson method (open technique)

b) Trocar with optical obturator

c) Veress needle (closed technique)

> Because of the large variety of trocars available and the resulting variety of methods of introducing the trocars, follow their individual instruction manuals!

> Note the following special features when creating the pneumoperitoneum in laparoscopic obesity surgery:
> - The thickness of the abdominal wall may require a larger incision, which may make gas-proof placement of the Hasson trocar difficult (→ p. 26, IIa)!
> - Use of an optical obturator in the trocar has proven to be helpful in obesity surgery (→ p. 27, IIb)!
> - Select the access of the Veress needle in the left abdomen in order to minimize the injury risk of patients with hepatomegaly (→ p. 28, IIc)!
> - The resting intra-abdominal pressure is often increased up to 8–9 mmHg!

CREATING THE PNEUMOPERITONEUM

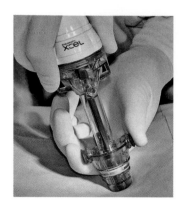

a) Hasson method (open technique)

Size 11 scalpel
Scissors
2 surgical forceps
2 Langenbeck hooks
2 retaining sutures (2–0)
Purse-string suture (2–0)
Hasson trocar (10/12 mm)

In obese patients, the use of the Hasson technique can be very difficult or even impossible!

Incise the skin about 18 cm below the xiphoid and 1–2 fingers paramedian on the left, making a 1.5–2 cm skin incision.

Ensure that the skin incision is the correct length:
• **An incision that is too small can make the insertion of the trocars much more difficult. If the skin around the trocar then suffers increased tension, this may lead to skin necrosis!**
• **An incision that is too large can result in gas loss and trocar dislocation (→ p. 60, V-5b)!**

Separate the subcutaneous fat with the scissors or bluntly with the finger tip as far as the rectus abdominis muscle. Use two Langenbeck hooks to expose the fascia of the anterior rectus sheath.

Then insert two 2–0 stay sutures on the fascia of the anterior rectus sheath and lift the fascia upwards by pulling on the sutures.

Use a scalpel to open the fascia between the two stay sutures over a distance of 1.5 cm. Then spread the rectus abdominis muscle as far as the posterior rectus sheath.

To expose the fascia of the posterior rectus sheath, retract the rectus abdominis muscle with its anterior sheath by repositioning the Langenbeck hooks.

Now lift the peritoneum with the surgical forceps and incise it with the scissors over a length of about 1–1.5 cm. Check for the presence of close adhesions by inserting a finger into the incision site and palpating over the entire 360° circumference of the site.

Place a purse-string suture around the peritoneal incision and introduce the blunt Hasson trocar through the incision into the free abdominal cavity.

Secure the trocar with the two previously placed stay sutures by tying them around the wings of the trocar cone. Tighten the purse-string suture around the Hasson trocar.

Connect the CO_2 supply tube to the trocar, remove the obturator, and insufflate the gas until the preselected maximum pressure is reached.

Alternative: It is possible to perform an open technique without using a Hasson trocar. After incising the fascia of the posterior rectus sheath and the peritoneum, place a blunt probe through the incision in the free abdominal cavity, using it as a support for the placement of the trocar for the scope under visual control.

b) Trocar with optical obturator

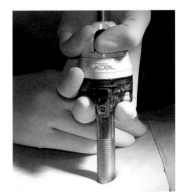

Size 11 scalpel
Trocar with optical obturator
Scope (0°)

Incise the skin about 15 cm below the xiphoid and 1–2 fingers paramedian on the left, making a 1–1.5 cm skin incision.

> **Ensure that the skin incision is the correct length:**
> • An incision that is too small can make the insertion of the trocars much more difficult. If the skin around the trocar then suffers increased tension, this may lead to skin necrosis!
> • An incision that is too large can result in gas loss and trocar dislocation (→ p. 60, V-5b)!

Insert the scope into the optical obturator located in the trocar and lock the scope-locking cam. Set the focus on the tip of the trocar. Turn the optic to have best exposure of the tip.

Place the transparent conical tip into the incision. Now carefully push the different layers of the abdominal wall tangentially parallel to the muscle fibers apart by applying light pressure and using to-and-fro rotating movements of the blunt obturator tip. The special construction of the obturator allows the layers to be identified before they are pushed apart.

Perform this tissue separation and the final perforation of the peritoneum under constant vision.

> **When inserting the trocar, take care**
> • to go in perpendicular to the abdominal wall,
> • to support the trocar with the hand, and
> • not to use excessive force in order to avoid blood vessel and organ injuries in the event of loss of resistance (→ p. 59, V-2; V-3)!

Finally, remove the scope together with the obturator from the trocar.

Connect the CO_2 supply tube to the trocar and insufflate the gas until the preselected maximum pressure is reached.

CREATING THE PNEUMOPERITONEUM

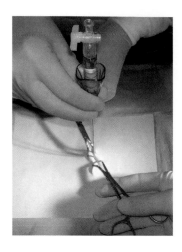

c) Veress needle (closed technique)

Insertion of the Veress needle and the first trocar are the most dangerous moments in minimally invasive surgery, as the insertion is done "blind". There are many reported cases of major injuries to the aorta and the iliac artery caused by the use of the Veress needle!

Size 11 scalpel
2 Backhaus clamps
Veress needle
10 ml syringe with NaCl solution
Trocar for the scope T1 (10/12 mm)

To minimize the risk of injury that may be caused by the Veress needle, in obese patients always select the access for the Veress needle in the left upper abdomen, subcostally in the midclavicular line, because of the usually existing hepatomegaly and the considerable amount of fatty tissue in these patients!

Patients who have undergone previous surgery carry a higher risk of having adhesions. In these patients, the Veress needle should be used with more caution!

Incise the skin about 18 cm below the xiphoid and 1–2 fingers paramedian on the left, making a 1–1.5 cm skin incision.

With the help of the assistant, elevate the abdominal wall with two Backhaus clamps, and carefully insert the Veress needle vertically, with your hand supported above the skin incision. The penetration of the abdominal wall layers by the Veress needle can be felt or even heard.

Alternative: Perform a blunt dissection of subcutaneous fat. Insert a Kocher clamp into the abdominal fascia and pull the abdominal wall with maximum strength.

When inserting the Veress needle, take care
• to go in perpendicular to the abdominal wall (→ p. 60, V-5a),
• to support the hand holding the needle, and
• not to use excessive force in order to avoid blood vessel and organ injuries in the event of loss of resistance (→ p. 59, V-2; V-3)!

Check the correct position of the Veress needle by applying the following obligatory safety tests:

Aspiration test
Attach a 10 ml syringe filled with NaCl solution to the Veress needle. It should be possible to aspirate air as a sign that the intra-abdominal position is correct.

Injection test
Inject NaCl solution through the Veress needle into the abdominal cavity. This can be done easily if it is in the correct position. Increased resistance of the syringe plunger indicates a possible incorrect position of the Veress needle.

Alternative: When using the ENDOPATH® Ultra Veress Insufflation Needle, Ethicon Endo-Surgery, the valve is opened to perform the injection test, whereupon the NaCl solution is released into the abdominal cavity if the Veress needle is in the correct position. In addition, the red marker ball drops down, indicating that NaCl solution is being released into the abdominal cavity.

Rotation test

Carefully rotate the slightly tilted needle inside the abdominal cavity. If the needle can be rotated freely, adhesions in close proximity are unlikely.

Slurp test

Notice that the slurp test is hardly feasible in case of pronounced obesity!

Apply one drop of NaCl solution onto the cone of the Veress needle, placing it convex on the opening. Now pull up the abdominal wall, making sure not to fix the Veress needle with your hand. Elevating the abdominal wall will create a partial vacuum, which in turn will cause the drop of NaCl to be sucked into the abdominal cavity, provided the Veress needle is correctly placed. A substantial vacuum will cause an additional "slurping" sound to be heard at the cone of the Veress needle.

If the safety tests indicate that the Veress needle has been placed correctly, attach the gas supply tube.

Excessively high intra-abdominal resting pressure and no flow indicate that the tip of the Veress needle is obstructed, e.g. by the greater omentum (→ **p. 59, V-3a**). In this case, perform the following test:

Manometer test

In order to release the Veress needle, manually lift up the abdominal wall. This should result in an obvious pressure drop. If this is not the case, remove the Veress needle and then place it again.

Notice that in obese patients the resting intra-abdominal pressure is often increased up to 8–9 mmHg!

Insufflate the CO_2 until the preselected maximum pressure is reached. After that, remove the Veress needle from the skin incision.

To be sure that the Veress needle has been placed correctly, check for an adequate flow during the CO_2 insufflation and an appropriate increase in pressure on the insufflator!

Now place the trocar for the scope in the skin incision about 18 cm below the xiphoid and 1–2 fingers paramedian on the left. To do so use either

• a trocar with a sharp tip (10/12 mm) or
• a trocar with optical obturator.

When inserting the trocar, take care
• to go in perpendicular to the abdominal wall,
• to support the trocar with the hand, and
• not to use excessive force in order to avoid blood vessel and organ injuries in the event of loss of resistance (→ p. 59, V-2; V-3)!

PLACING THE WORKING TROCARS

Trocar for the scope T1 (10/12 mm)
Working trocar T2 (5 mm or 10/12 mm; depending on the liver retracting device)
Working trocar T3 (10/12 mm)
Working trocar T4 (10/12 mm)
Size 11 scalpel
Reducer caps, if necessary

Insert the scope into the trocar (T1).

Then position the patient in a reverse Trendelenburg position in order that the small intestine slides into the lower abdomen by gravity and to obtain an optimal view of the operating field (→ p. 24, I).

Perform a diagnostic laparoscopy to make sure that there are no pathological changes and/or injuries which might require an alteration of the operative strategy or even prevent continuation of the operation (→ **p. 59, V-2; V-3**).

The liver is retracted through the trocar T2. The positions of the other working trocars depend on the operative site and are therefore established after the liver retracting device has been inserted.

Place the working trocar T2 subxiphoidal or on the right subcostally, approximately in the midclavicular line. Choose the working trocar site T2 by palpating the abdominal wall under vision and use diaphanoscopy to ensure that no major cutaneous vessels will be injured when the trocar is inserted (→ **p. 59, V-1; V-2**).

T2: In the right upper abdomen subcostal midclavicular line or subxiphoidal (depending on liver size and liver retracting device)

Incise the skin with a scalpel according to the trocar diameter: about 1 cm when using a 5 mm trocar and about 1.5 cm with a 10/12 mm trocar. Now insert the working trocar under vision.

Ensure that the skin incision is the right size!

When placing the trocar make sure that it points exactly towards the operating field, as later corrections will not be possible.

When placing the trocar, take care
• **to insert the trocar under vision to avoid injuries (→ p. 59, V-2; V-3), and**
• **to point the trocar exactly towards the operating field, as later corrections will be difficult, if not impossible in obese abdominal walls!**

After inserting the liver retracting device, an unrestricted view of the operating field should be guaranteed. Then fix the liver retracting device to the fixation arm.

Place the liver retracting device carefully and always under vision, as in obese patients the texture of the liver is often fat, which increases the vulnerability of the tissue (→ p. 60, V-3d)!

Choose the working trocar sites T3 and T4 depending on the operative site, roughly in a half-moon around the trocar for the scope, and by palpating the abdominal wall under vision. Use diaphanoscopy to ensure that no major cutaneous vessels will be injured when the trocar is inserted (→ **p. 59, V-1; V-2**).

> **T3:** In the right epigastrium, 1–2 fingers paramedian on the right, one hand's breadth above the optic trocar (T1)
>
> **T4:** In the left epigastrium, left midclavicular line one hand's breadth above the optic trocar (T1); T1, T3 and the xyphoid should form an equilateral triangle

Insert the trocars according to the above description for T2, starting with the skin incisions.

> **When placing the trocars, take care**
> • to insert the trocars under vision to avoid injuries (→ p. 59, V-2; V-3),
> • to point the trocars exactly towards the operating field, as later corrections will be difficult, if not impossible in obese abdominal walls,
> • to place additional trocars at any time to gain optimal working conditions, and
> • to place the trocars with a minimum distance of 10 cm between them in order to avoid interference of camera and instruments!

Remove the obturators from the trocars and attach the reducer caps to T3 and T4, if necessary.

> **Alternative:** If the liver is greatly enlarged, requiring the use of another liver retracting device, insert an additional trocar (T5). The location of the trocar depends on the intra-operative site.

> **Alternative:** Some surgeons prefer to place an additional trocar for the assistant in the left lateral abdomen.

> There are many ways to position the trocars. We prefer the placement described above, but it should be the surgeon's choice!

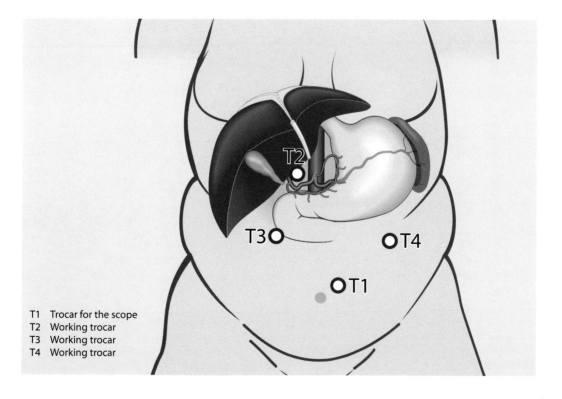

T1 Trocar for the scope
T2 Working trocar
T3 Working trocar
T4 Working trocar

01 **Exploring the abdominal cavity**

02 **Identifying the anatomical landmarks**

03 **Dissecting the greater curvature towards the pylorus**

04 **Dissecting the greater curvature towards the angle of His**

05 **Dissecting the posterior gastric wall**

06 **Calibrating the gastric pouch**

07 **Creating the gastric sleeve**

08 **Oversewing the staple line**

09 **Testing the stomach for leaks**

10 **Removing the resected stomach**

11 **Finishing the operation**

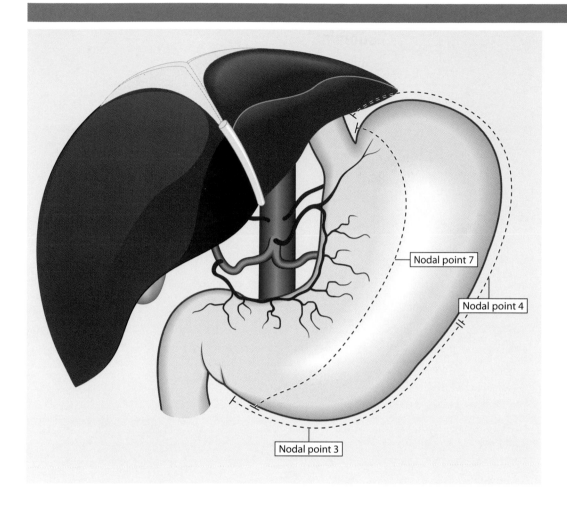

Nodal point 7

Nodal point 4

Nodal point 3

1 Exploring the abdominal cavity

T1   Scope
T2   Liver retracting device
T3   Atraumatic grasping forceps, if necessary
T4   Harmonic® shears or curved scissors, if necessary

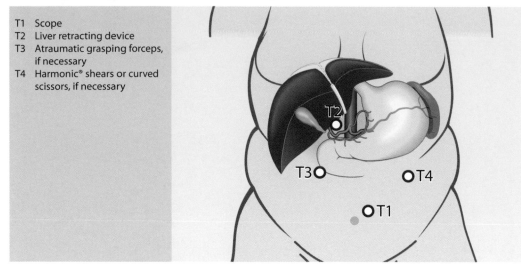

Examine the abdominal cavity carefully by inspecting it in a clockwise direction. Due to obesity a thorough inspection of the structures in the pelvis might be difficult.

- Pelvis: dome of the bladder, pouch of Douglas, the internal hernial orifices, and the uterus and adnexa in women
- Cecum with appendix
- Ascending colon
- Right upper abdomen: liver and gallbladder, right colonic flexure
- Greater omentum
- Transverse colon
- Left upper abdomen: stomach and spleen, splenic flexure
- Descending colon
- Sigmoid colon
- Jejunum and ileum

Look particularly for adhesions, erythema, vascular injections, serous fluid, pus, tumors and peritoneal carcinosis.

> **If a tumor or infection is found during the exploration, performing the gastric sleeve is contraindicated!**

Particularly check the trocar incision sites for adhesions and possible bleedings. Change the scope position, if necessary (→ **p. 59, V-1; V-2**).

Divide any adhesions in the operating field using sharp dissection (→ **p. 59, V-1**).

> **Divide any adhesions to organs promptly in order to avoid injuries (→ p. 59, V-3)!**

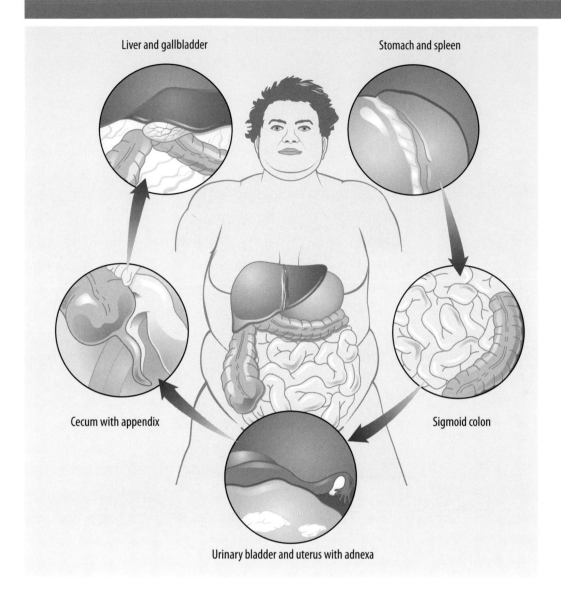

Liver and gallbladder

Stomach and spleen

Cecum with appendix

Sigmoid colon

Urinary bladder and uterus with adnexa

2 Identifying the anatomical landmarks

T1 Scope
T2 Liver retracting device
T3 Atraumatic grasping forceps
T4 Harmonic® shears, curved dissector or curved scissors, if necessary

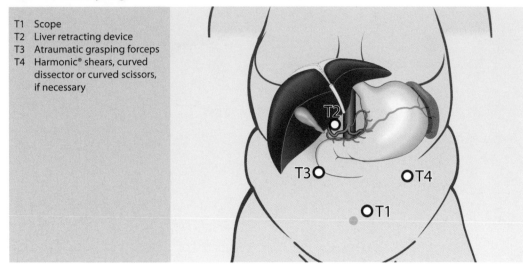

Identify the following anatomical landmarks:

Upper abdomen:
- Caudate and left liver lobe with falciform ligament
- Lesser omentum with hepatogastric ligament
- Left gastric artery, if possible
- Gastro-esophageal junction
- Stomach: lesser and greater curvature, angle of His and pylorus
- Spleen with gastrophrenic ligament

In case of fat accumulations in the subcardiac region of the stomach and at the gastro-esophageal junction, use a dissector or sharp dissection to remove them in order to ensure an optimal view of the operating field.

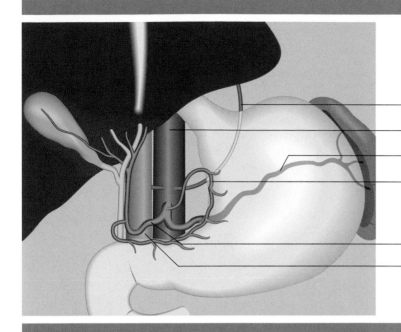

Inferior phrenic artery

Aorta

Splenic artery

Left gastric artery

Common hepatic artery

Vena cava

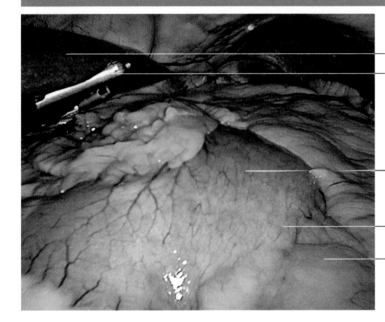

Liver

Liver retracting device

Stomach

Greater curvature of the stomach

Greater omentum

3 Dissecting the greater curvature towards the pylorus

T1   Scope
T2   Liver retracting device
T3   Atraumatic grasping forceps
T4   Harmonic® shears

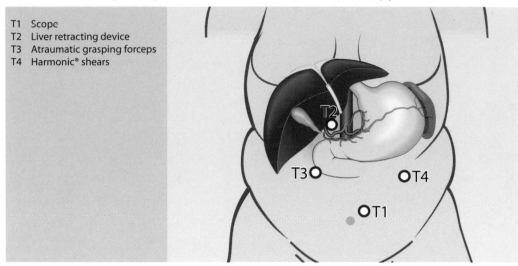

Grasp the lower part of the corpus with an atraumatic forceps (T3) and lift it up.

Insert the Harmonic® shears through T4 and open the gastrocolic ligament at the middle of the greater curvature.

Dissect the greater curvature towards the pylorus (T4). Dissect near the gastric wall and take care not to injure the gastroepiploic vessels.

> **Make sure to dissect close to the gastric wall and take care not to injure the gastroepiploic vessels to avoid severe bleedings (→ p. 59, V-2).**

Identify the pylorus and stop the dissection at a distance of 1–2 cm to the pylorus. However make sure that the stomach is mobilized in the area of the first endoscopic linear cutter placement.

> **Take care not to injure the antrum wall, duodenum, or pancreatic capsule during the dissection with Harmonic® shears (→ p. 59, V-3).**

> **Alternative: It is also possible to dissect towards the angle of His before dissecting towards the pylorus.**

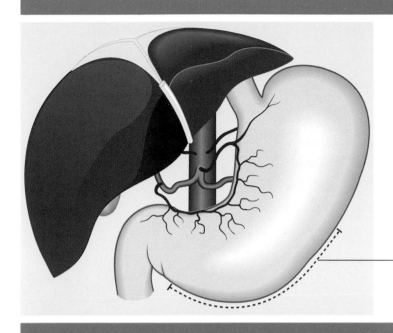

Dissection line

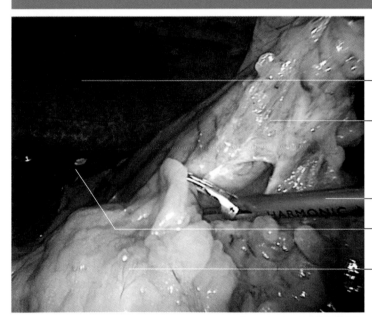

Liver

Greater curvature of the stomach

Dissection device (Harmonic® shears)

Liver retracting device

Greater omentum

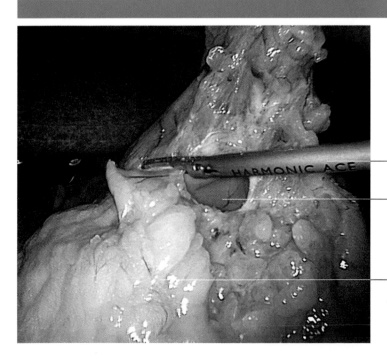

Dissection device (Harmonic® shears)

Posterior wall of the stomach

Greater omentum

4 Dissecting the greater curvature towards the angle of His

T1   Scope
T2   Liver retracting device
T3   Atraumatic grasping forceps
T4   Harmonic® shears

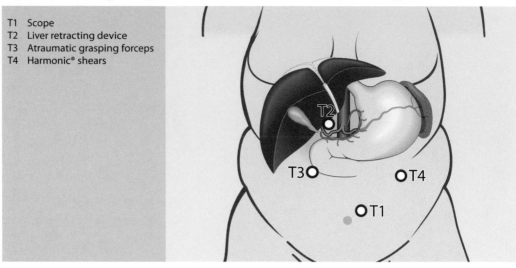

Grasp the stomach with an atraumatic forceps (T3) and draw it laterally to the right.

> **Be careful not to tear too much at the stomach wall to avoid injuries of the splenic capsule or vessels (→ p. 59, V-3).**

Dissect the greater curvature with Harmonic shears (T4) towards the angle of His and stay close to the gastric wall.

> **Take care to dissect close to the gastric wall in order not to injure the spleen, esophagus or diaphragm during the dissection with Harmonic® shears (→ p. 59, V-3).**

Expose the spleen and transect the short gastric vessels.

Then grasp the fundus (T3) and push it downward to the right to expose the left crus of the diaphragm.

Check for hiatal hernia (→ p. 60, V-4).

> **Alternative: If necessary place an additional trocar (T5) in the left upper abdomen quadrant (2 cm subcostal with a minimum of 10 cm above T3). Insert the Harmonic® shears and continue the dissection of the greater curvature towards the angle of His.**

> **Alternative: Dissecting the angle of His before dissecting the short gastric vessels reduces the tension on the stomach and let the stomach slide towards the lower abdomen. This helps to obtain an optimal view of the operating field.**

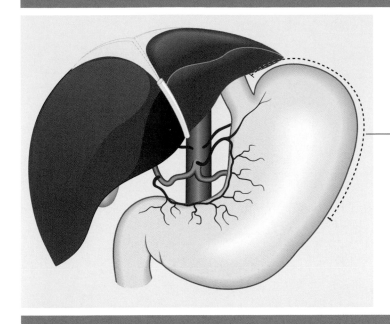

Dissection line

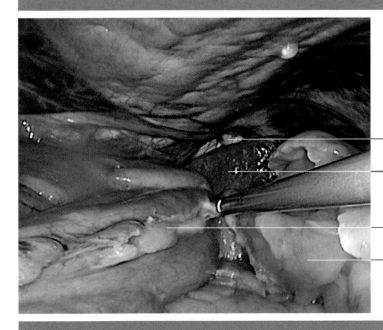

Diaphragm

Spleen

Greater curvature of the stomach

Greater omentum

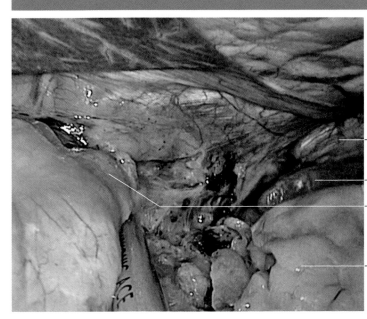

Diaphragm

Spleen

Greater curvature of the stomach

Greater omentum

NODAL POINTS

5 Dissecting the posterior gastric wall

T1   Scope
T2   Liver retracting device
T3   Atraumatic grasping forceps
T4   Harmonic® shears

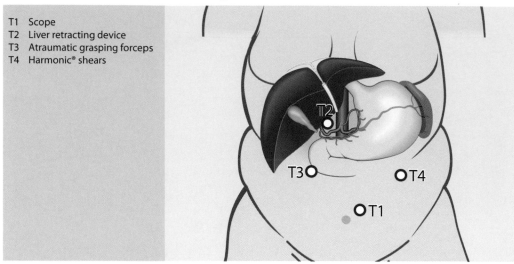

Grasp the gastric corpus with an atraumatic forceps (T3) and pull it laterally to the right.

Mobilize the posterior gastric wall with the Harmonic® shears (T4) and dissect any adhesions to the retroperitoneum to prevent dilatation of the sleeve, which usually occurs at the posterior gastric wall (→ **p. 68, appendices**).

> **Be careful not to injure the vascularisation of the lesser curvature, which can lead to necrosis of the remaining stomach (→ p. 69, appendices).**

Mobilize the stomach completely to assure proper linear cutter placement subsequently.

> **Prevent injuries of the pancreatic capsule during dissection by placing the inactive blade of the Harmonic® shears towards the fragile structures (→ p. 59, V-3).**

> **Alternative: Using an additional trocar can ease the entry of the greater sac. Grasp the gastrocolic ligament with an additional atraumatic forceps and pull it to the left.**

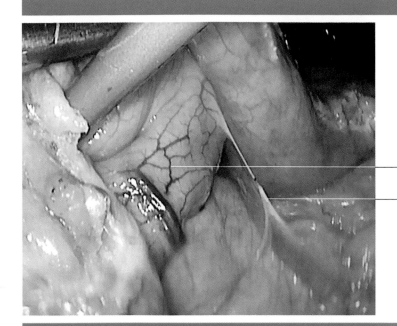

Posterior wall of the stomach

Adhesions

Mobilizing the posterior wall

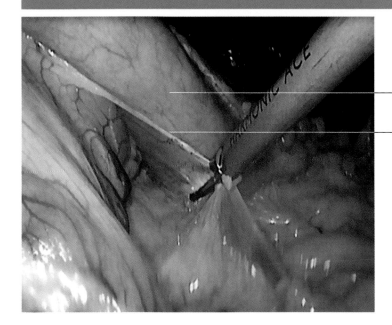

Posterior wall of the stomach

Adhesions

6 Calibrating the gastric pouch

T1   Scope
T2   Liver retracting device
T3   Atraumatic grasping forceps
T4   Atraumatic grasping forceps

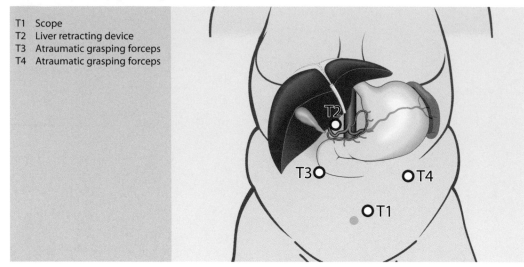

Grasp the fundus with an atraumatic forceps (T3) and stabilize the stomach.

Ask the anesthetist to insert a calibration tube with a size of 32–42 french transorally. Use an atraumatic forceps (T4) and help the anesthetist to guide down the bougie until the tip of the tube comes to lie in the antrum.

Instruct the anesthetist not to remove or displace the tube during the operation in order to avoid a too narrow sleeve or even a stenosis!

Create a pouch volume of 100–150 ml to achieve more lasting weight loss, if a stand-alone sleeve gastrectomy is planned. In a staged concept when a second intervention is planned, consider leaving a larger pouch volume.

Be careful not to leave too much stomach volume to prevent postoperative dilatation (→ p. 68, appendices). However, do not resect too much, as this may lead to postoperative reflux (→ p. 69, appendices).

Alternative: Instead of a calibration tube a gastroscope (9–10 mm) can be used. This assures a proper placement of the calibration tube and provides a visible control of the staple line and suture at the end of the procedure.

Cardia

Fundus

Body

Calibration tube

Antrum

Pylorus

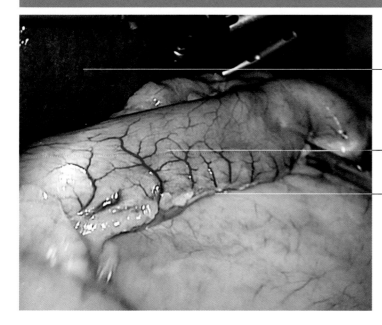

Placing the calibration tube

Liver

Stomach with calibration tube

Greater curvature

7 Creating the gastric sleeve

T1 Scope
T2 Liver retracting device
T3 Linear cutter, later atraumatic grasping forceps
T4 Atraumatic grasping forceps, later linear cutter

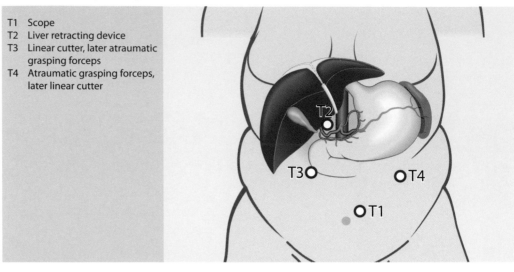

Instruct the anesthetist not to move the calibration tube while stapling in order to avoid a too narrow sleeve!

Grasp the fundus with an atraumatic forceps (T4) and pull it laterally to the left.

Insert the endoscopic linear cutter (T3) and place it at the antrum at a distance of 2–6 cm to the pylorus.

Note that there is still no consensus about the starting point of resection as each antrum has its individual size. The authors recommend stapling at a distance of 2–6 cm from the pylorus to avoid stapling into the pylorus!

Due to the thick antrum wall it is recommended to start with green cartridges (2.0 mm closed staple height).

Position the endoscopic linear cutter on the tissue, then close the instrument.

Before firing,
- **take care not to grasp too much tissue, as accumulation of tissue at the proximal end of the jaws may result an incomplete staple line (→ p. 67, appendices),**
- **make sure not to grasp the calibration tube itself with the endoscopic linear cutter,**
- **inspect the dorsal aspect of the gastric wall before firing to avoid any twisting or sacculations of the gastric wall (→ p. 68/69, appendices).**

Prior to firing, keep the jaws fully closed for about 15 seconds (or longer i.e. in redo cases with scar tissue). The accurate tissue compression minimizes the tissue liquid and ensures proper and safe staple line.

Fire the endoscopic linear cutter.

Open the jaws of the endoscopic linear cutter and remove the instrument for reloading.

Continue stapling the sleeve in a linear way at the left lateral side of the calibration tube parallel to the length of the greater curvature.

Due to different thickness of the stomach wall, use green cartridges (2.0 mm closed staple height) in the region of the pylorus and the antrum, gold cartridges (1.8 mm closed staple height) in the region of the body and blue cartridges (1.5 mm closed staple height) in the region of the fundus.

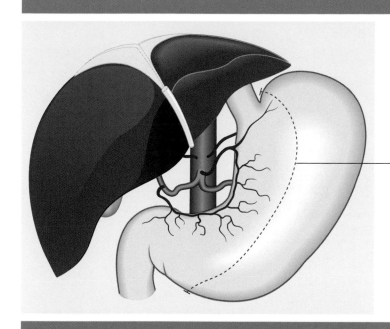

Staple line

First stapling of the linear cutter

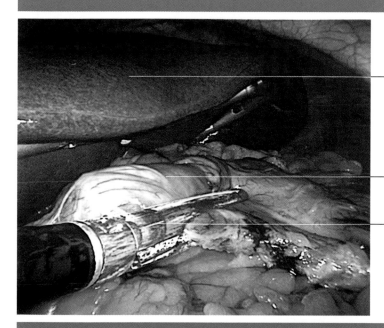

Liver

Stomach with calibration tube

Endoscopic linear cutter

Fourth firing with an articulating endoscopic linear stapler

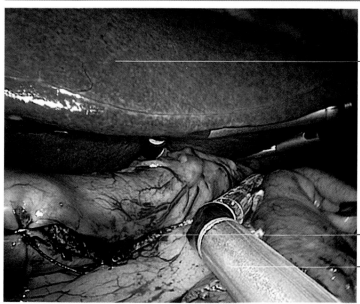

Liver

Staple line

Endoscopic linear cutter

7 Creating the gastric sleeve

T1   Scope
T2   Liver retracting device
T3   Linear cutter, later atraumatic grasping forceps
T4   Atraumatic grasping forceps, later linear cutter

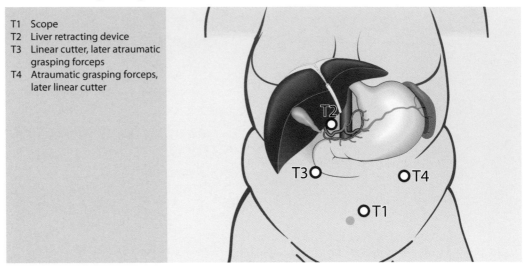

Take care to staple in a linear way at the left lateral side of the calibration tube (not dorsally or ventrally) and avoid twists or sacculations of the staple line. This may provoke torsion of the sleeve with functional stenosis, pseudodiverticulosis or kinking (→ p. 69, appendices).

Divide the stomach until the angle of His is reached. This enables a resection of the complete gastric fundus, which harbors the ghrelin-secreting cells of the stomach.

To resect all ghrelin-secreting cells take care to transect the complete fundus.

Take care not to staple into the esophagus (→ p. 59, V-3).

Remove the endoscopic linear cutter.

Alternative: Starting the oversewing of the antrum, while the linear stapler is being reloaded, can save time.

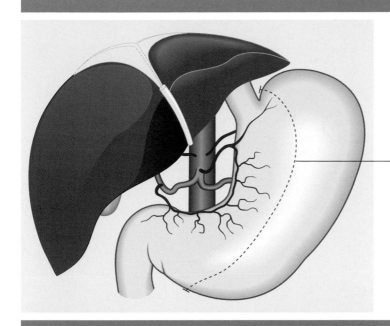

Staple line

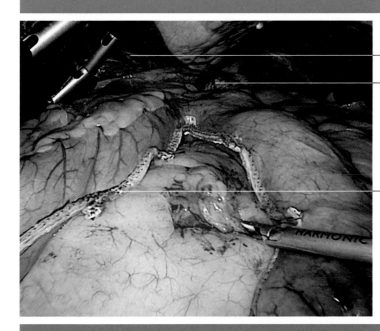

Liver

Diaphragm

Staple line

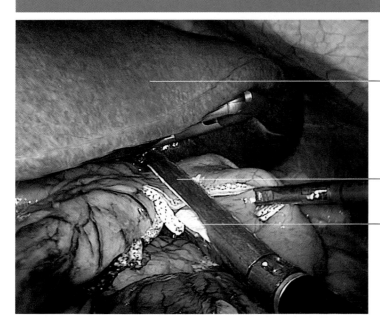

Liver

Endoscopic linear cutter

Staple line

8   Oversewing the staple line

T1   Scope
T2   Liver retracting device
T3   Atraumatic grasping forceps
T4   Needle holder

– absorbable sutures 1–0
   (e. g. Vicryl™)

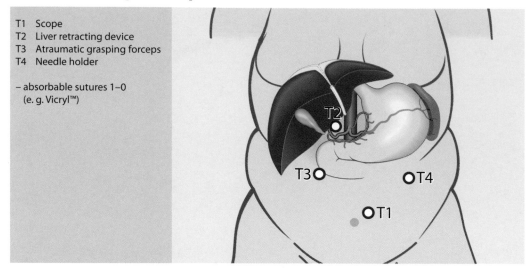

There is no strong evidence so far for the benefit of using buttress material or oversewing the staple line. The authors recommend oversewing the staple line, especially in the area of the strong antrum muscle and the angle of His, to reduce the risk of bleeding or leakage; it is also done to reshape the sleeve, e.g. if large portions of the dorsal gastric wall are left in place.

Oversew the antrum meticulously.

Grasp the distal part of the antrum with an atraumatic forceps (T3) and insert a needle holder with a 1–0 absorbable thread (e.g. Vicryl™) (T4).

Place as many Z- and one-stitch-sutures as you need to ensure a completely invaginated distal staple line.

> Make sure that the distal end of the staple line is completely invaginated.

Grasp the stomach with an atraumatic forceps in the angle of His region (T3) and oversew the proximal end of the staple line as described above.

> Especially the proximal and the distal end of the staple line carry a higher risk of staple line leakage (→ p. 67, appendices).

Complete the oversewing by placing Z-sutures running downwards from the angle of His, if necessary.

> Alternative: As far as can be judged from the literature, using buttress material might reduce the risk of postoperative bleedings. However, the proximal and distal ends of the staple line must be oversewn whether buttress material is used or not!

> Alternative: Oversew the staple line with single-layer sutures using absorbable suture clips (e.g. LAPRA-TY®). Using LAPRA-TY® provides the advantage of a re-adjustable suture which ensures a proper size and forming of the sleeve. Two or three sutures of 18–20 cm should be sufficient to oversew the staple line completely.

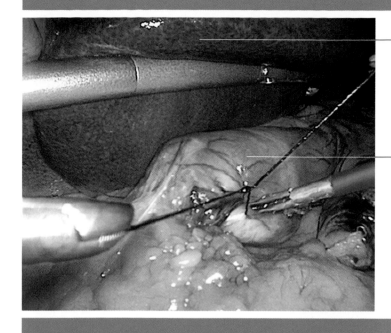

Liver

Antrum

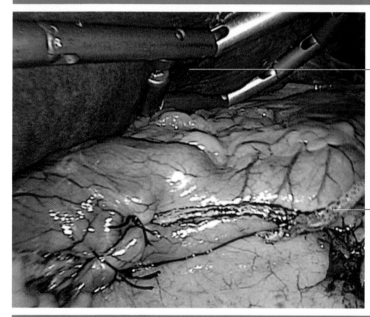

Liver

Staple line

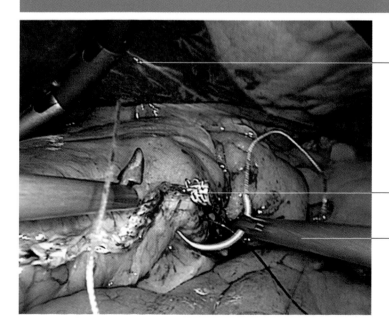

Liver

Staple line

Needle holder

9 Testing the stomach for leaks

T1   Scope
T2   Liver retracting device
T3   –
T4   Atraumatic grasping forceps

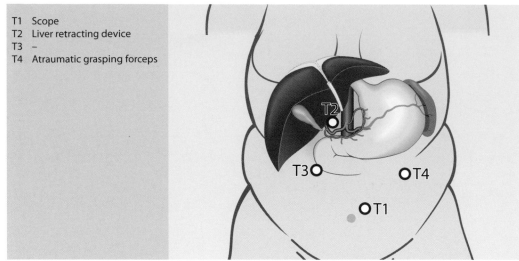

Insert an atraumatic instrument (T4) and occlude the gastric antrum.

Ask the anesthetist to pull back the calibration tube for 2 cm and to fill the tube with methylene blue solution until the stomach is stretched.

Watch for extravasation of dye while methylene blue is allowed to run into the pouch. Pay special attention to the proximal end of the staple line.

If no dye is monitored, the test is considered negative (→ **p. 61, V-7**).

Ask the anesthetist to suck off the liquid from the pouch and to measure the volume of the methylene blue solution. Then have him remove the calibration tube.

Alternative: Instead of the methylene blue test an air leakage test can be performed. Insert an atraumatic instrument (T4) and occlude the proximal jejunum. Ask the anesthetist to fill the calibration tube with air. Insert an irrigation device and supply saline solution into the abdominal cavity (T3). Watch for upcoming bubbles while air is allowed to flow into the pouch. Pay special attention to the proximal end of the staple line. If no bubbles are monitored, the test is considered negative.

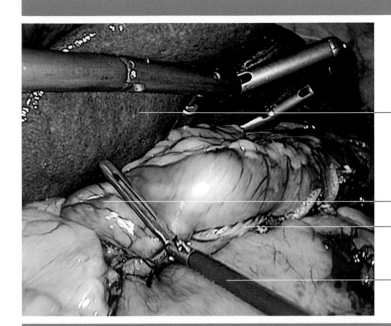

Liver

Antrum

Staple line

Atraumatic instrument

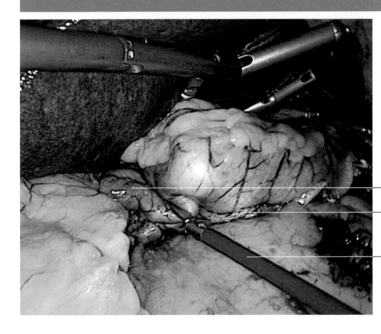

Antrum

Staple line

Atraumatic instrument

10 Removing the resected stomach

T1   Scope
T2   Liver retracting device
T3   Atraumatic grasping forceps
T4   Needle holder, atraumatic grasping forceps

– Retrieval pouch
– Surgical forceps, if necessary

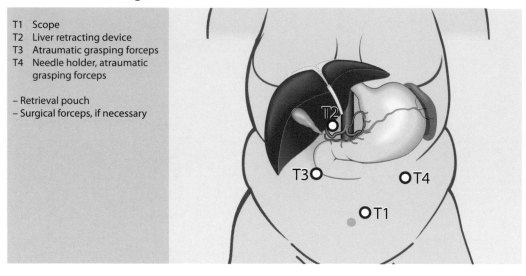

Grasp the resected stomach with an atraumatic forceps (T3).

Insert a needle holder with a 1-0 thread (T4) and place a holding thread at one end of the resected stomach.

Insert a plastic retrieval pouch through the working port (T4) and grasp it with an atraumatic forceps (T3).

Grasp the resected stomach with an atraumatic forceps (T4) and put it into the retrieval pouch.

Leave the holding thread outside and close the retrieval pouch.

Grasp the thread and pull on it to orientate the specimen in a sagital direction. This facilitates the retrieval.

> **Use always a plastic retrieval pouch to prevent abdominal wall infections. In case of a specimen rupture it also protects the subcutaneous tissue and facilitates the removal of the stomach.**

Remove the instrument and the trocar from T4. Luxate the opening of the retrieval pouch through the incision of T4. If necessary use a forceps. Open the bag from outside and grasp the holding thread. Pull on it and extract the specimen from the retrieval pouch. Enlarge the size of the trocar incision digitally, if necessary.

> **Alternative: Enlarge the size of the trocar incision (T4) with a scalpel if there are still difficulties in removing the specimen.**

> **Alternative: Measure the volume of the resected stomach by filling it with physiological saline. Check the resected stomach for leaks (→ p. 61, V-8). A resected stomach volume of less than 500 ml is considered to be insufficient and requires revision!**

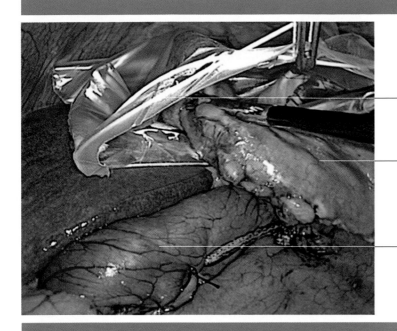

Retrieval bag

Resected stomach

Created sleeve

Resected stomach

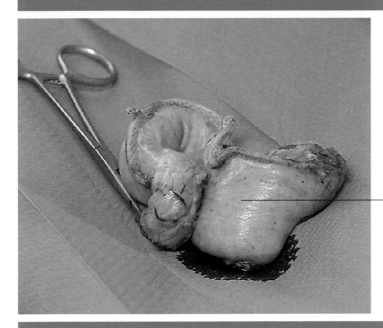

Resected stomach

Measuring the volume of the resected stomach

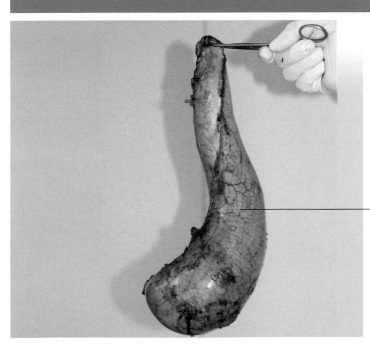

Resected stomach

11 **Finishing the operation**

T1   Scope
T2   Liver retracting device
T3   Atraumatic grasping forceps
T4   –

– Surgical forceps
– Needle holder
– Suture scissors
– 2 Langenbeck hooks
– Fascia sutures 2–0 absorbable, polyfilament
– Subcutaneous sutures 3–0 absorbable, polyfilament, if necessary
– Skin sutures 4–0 or 5–0 absorbable, monofilament or a skin stapler
– Dressings

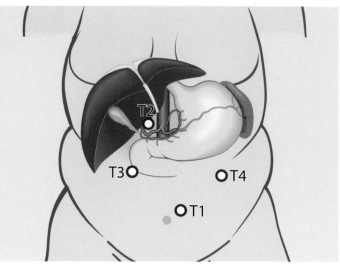

Insert a silicone drain through T4. Grasp it with an atraumatic forceps (T3) and place it beyond the posterior wall of the stomach. Fix the silicone drain with a suture and attach a drainage bag.

Remove the liver retracting device and the working trocar (T2, T3) carefully under vision.

Check the trocar incisions with regard to possible bleeding (→ **p. 59, V-2**).

Remove the scope (T1) and open the valve on the trocar for deflation. Then remove the trocar for the scope.

Close all incisions and cover the wounds with sterile dressings following disinfection.

> **Alternative: Instead of skin sutures and dressings Dermabond® (Ethicon Products) can be used to close the skin incisions.**

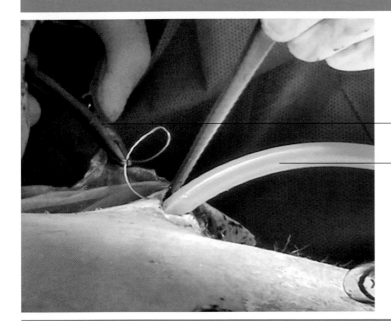

Needle holder

Drainage

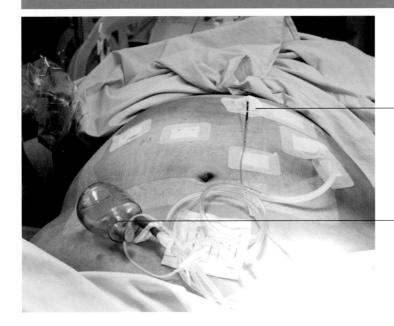

Dressings

Drainage

MANAGEMENT OF DIFFICULT SITUATIONS AND COMPLICATIONS

In principle, the decision to proceed to laparotomy should be made too early rather than too late! In obese patients, however, the possibility of other trocar positions should be considered before converting to a conventional operation in order to gain a better view! Convert immediately if the situation cannot be controlled laparoscopically!

1 Adhesions

Separate adhesions using the Harmonic® shears or curved scissors as close to the abdominal wall as possible and as much as needed to get free access to the left upper quadrant.

2 Blood vessel injuries

a) Diffuse bleeding/bleeding from minor vessels

Coagulate the bleeding vessel with the Harmonic® shears, electrocautery or argon laser beamer. If this does not terminate the bleeding, place a clip on the bleeding vessel or oversew it.

Stop any bleeding close to the gastric wall ideally with the HF electrode or the ultrasonic device or with an atraumatic transfixing suture.

b) Bleeding from major vessels

If large vessels such as the aorta, portal vein, or vena cava are injured during the operation, open the abdomen immediately for vascular surgical treatment of the injury!

3 Organ injuries

In case of injuries where the extent cannot be determined with certainty, open the abdominal cavity for open management of the injury.

a) Greater omentum

Injury of the greater omentum can occur when the Veress needle is inserted too deeply and/or without elevation of the abdominal wall. All the safety tests may be positive, so that the complication can be identified only when the trocar for the scope and the scope are inserted.

Manage any bleeding that occurs with the Harmonic® shears. If, as a result of the insertion, the greater omentum is inflated like a tent, withdraw the trocar for the scope as far as the peritoneal margin and tap the abdomen with the flat hand. The omentum should then separate from the inside of the abdominal wall and collapse.

b) Esophagus

Injury to the esophagus is a very serious complication. Oversew the injury very carefully and then finish the operation without creating a gastric sleeve.

In case of an injury to the esophagus oversew the injury very carefully and do not perform a gastric sleeve procedure!

c) Stomach

Perform gastroscopy to confirm a gastric injury and examine precisely where the lesion is located.

Oversew the lesion carefully with 1-0 absorbable material. Suturing of the defect can be done laparoscopically or in a conventional operation, depending on the extent of the lesion.

In case of staple line bleeding do not coagulate, as coagulation carries the risk of subsequent necrosis. Use clips or a suture to achieve safe hemostasis.

d) Liver

Manage minor bleeding from the liver by brief compression with a swab or point contact with the Harmonic® shears or argon laser beamer.

In the case of major hemorrhaging that can still be controlled laparoscopically, apply a hemostyptic.

e) Spleen

Bleeding from the spleen is ideally treated with the Harmonic® shears. Alternatively, apply a hemostyptic or perform laparotomy, depending on the extent of the injury. Laparotomy is the exception.

f) Bowel

Bowel injuries are usually caused by instruments, especially by the Veress needle. Undissected adhesions can also be a cause of bowel injuries.

Manage bowel injuries by laparoscopic oversewing. If sufficient closure of the injury is not guaranteed, perform laparotomy. Irrigate the operating field gently with an antiseptic solution in order to reduce the risk of infection. As bowel resections always require a systemic antibiotic (single dose), the patient should already have antibiotic coverage (→ p. 19, I).

g) Pancreas

Manage minor bleeding from the pancreas by brief compression with a swab or point contact with Harmonic® shears.

In the case of major hemorrhaging that can still be controlled laparoscopically, apply a hemostyptic.

4   Hiatal hernia

Check for a hiatal hernia and if present, reduce it and close the phrenic pillars with sutures.

5   Preperitoneal air emphysema

a) Veress needle

If emphysema has occurred because of an incorrectly placed needle, remove the needle and reinsert it as previously described (→ p. 28, IIc). Ensure particularly that the angle of insertion is vertical and that the abdominal wall is lifted.

b) Trocar

Withdrawing a trocar so far that its opening comes to lie in front of the peritoneum is another cause of emphysema.

In this case, under direct vision, push the trocar back into the correct position through the existing incision.

6 Losing a swab in the abdominal cavity

After losing a swab, fix the trocar in its last position and, under vision, look for the swab where it was lost, using an atraumatic grasping forceps.

Do not change the patient's position, and do not irrigate the abdominal cavity!

If necessary, search for the swab with the C-arm or perform a laparotomy to retrieve the swab.

Do not give up searching until the swab is found!

7 Positive methylene blue leak test

If the leak test is positive, the defect must be repaired. Oversew the leakage using Z- and One-Stitch-sutures. Repeat the leak test.

8 Leakage from the resected stomach

If a leak in the staple line of the resected stomach occurs while the volume of the specimen is being measured, oversew the corresponding area of the gastric sleeve.

APPENDICES

Anatomical variations

Sample operation note

Postoperative management

a) Analgesia
b) Mobilization
c) Nutrition
d) Diagnostics
e) Medication
f) Discharge

Management of postoperative complications

a) Sleeve stenosis
b) Staple line leakage
c) Fistula
d) Sleeve dilatation
e) Gastroesophageal reflux
f) Sleeve necrosis
g) Functional stenosis due to torsion of the sleeve (kinking)

Bibliography

Keywords

Editors

Assistants

Titles available

APPENDICES

Anatomical variations

Accessory hepatic artery

In about 20 % of cases an accessory hepatic artery may be present in the region of the pars flaccida. Be aware of this possible anatomical variation during manipulation.

Sample operation note

Date:	Operating surgeon:
Patient's name:	Assistant:
Operation diagnosis: Morbid adipositas	Scrub nurse:
Operation: Laparoscopic Sleeve Gastrectomy	Anesthetist:

Patient under general anesthesia, placed in lithotomy position with adequate padding. Skin disinfection and sterile draping, followed by a skin incision 18 cm below the xiphoid and 1–2 fingers paramedian on the left.

The Veress needle is inserted transmuscularly through the incision and the usual safety tests are carried out. Pneumoperitoneum is then established with a pressure of 15 mmHg.

A 12 mm trocar for the scope is placed through this incision and the scope is brought into the abdomen. The patient is then placed in a reverse Trendelenburg position. A 360° view reveals no pathological changes and/or injuries. Under direct visualization a 5 mm trocar is placed in the right upper abdomen and the liver retracting device is inserted and fixed with the self-retainer.

Then two 12 mm trocars are placed in the right and left epigastrium, respectively, under vision.

The omentum is separated from the stomach using Harmonic® shears. Starting in the middle of the greater curvature, the greater omentum is dissected towards the pylorus for a distance of approximately 2 cm. The dissection is continued towards the angle of His. The left and right crus of the diaphragm are exposed. The dorsal gastric wall is completely freed by dissecting all adhesions.

The gastric calibration tube is inserted by the anesthetist and is advanced into the stomach down to the antrum.

The gastric sleeve is created using the Echelon Flex™ Endopath® stapler, Ethicon Endo-Surgery (60 mm). The first firing (green cartridges) is placed in the antrum 2–6 cm proximal to the pylorus. The staple line is continued proximally along the gastric calibration tube. In the corpus gold cartridges and in the fundus blue cartridges are used. The staple line is completed at the angle of His. Care is taken not to staple into the esophagus.

The staple line is carefully oversewn with 2 running sutures PDS 3/0. A drain is placed behind the stomach. A stay suture is placed on the tip of the specimen, and the specimen is put into the retrieval bag. The bag is removed with the help of the stay suture.

The gastric sleeve is tested for leaks, and the gastric calibration tube is then removed by the anesthetist.

Following inspection of the operating field, the trocars are removed. The incisions are closed and covered with sterile dressings.

Postoperative management

a) Analgesia

Take care to give adequate pain medication for fast recovery of the patient.

On day of operation give opioids as needed by the patient. From the first postoperative day prescription of simple analgesia (NSAIDs) is sufficient in most cases.

> **Alternative: Infiltrating the trocar sites with carbostesine/adrenaline before incising reduces the need for analgetics.**

b) Mobilization

Depending on anesthetic aftereffects and circulatory stability, mobilize the patient as soon as possible postoperatively. Try to do so on the evening of the operation.

c) Nutrition

Reintroduction of food differs from hospital to hospital. Our recommendation is the following:

Day of operation and first postoperative day: Nourish the patient parenterally.

> **Alternative: Some hospitals perform an upper gastrointestinal (GI) X-ray series with Gastrografin on a routine basis. They start nourishing the patient with clear liquids, if the findings are inconspicuous. If a prolonged emptying of the sleeve occurs, they add a prokinetic pharmaceutical to the medication.**

Second postoperative day: Practice gradual reintroduction of food with four cups of tea.

Third postoperative day: Start with mashed food.

Fourth postoperative day: The reintroduction of solid food should take place with the assistance of a nutritionist.

Especially during the middle to long-term postoperative observation of the patient take, watch for potential deficiency of trace elements or vitamins (i.e. vitamin B_{12}). If it occurs give the patient the necessary food supplements.

d) Diagnostics

Take blood samples and control the vital signs regularly. This enables you to detect a tachycardia quite early. Tachycardia predominates as the first sign of sepsis in postoperative bariatric patients.

In obese patients the symptoms of sepsis such as abdominal pain, fever, or leukocytosis often occur later than they generally do in patients with normal BMI.

e) Medication

Medication should consist of gastric acid inhibitors (PPI) for about 2–4 weeks and low-molecular-weight heparin for anticoagulation combined with graded elastic compression stockings minimally during hospitalization up to 4 weeks. If the patient is known to have diabetes mellitus, measure the blood glucose level continuously, sometimes it is necessary to reduce the required insulin units.

f) Discharge

Discharge the patient between the fourth and seventh day. Prior to discharge make sure that the patient is mobilized, has passed urine, is free of pain, and is tolerating soft foods.

Perform complete follow-ups at 1, 6 and 12 months postoperatively and annually thereafter.

Management of postoperative complications

a) Sleeve stenosis

Sleeve stenosis can happen immediately after the operation or in the course of time. Stenosis and suture line insufficiency can occur in combination, as the distally located stenosis can cause an insufficiency in the fundus. They often occur after operations in which a too small sleeve was created.

In case of stenosis place a stent for 4–6 weeks. If stenosis recurs, it may be necessary to perform a gastric bypass operation.

> **There is no indication for balloon dilatation, as it carries an increased risk of damaging the staple line.**

b) Staple line leakage

Staple line leakage can occur as an early or a late postoperative complication. It can be caused by repetitive vomiting. Typically, the first symptom is a rapid pulse.

> **Tachycardia exceeding 120 bpm in the early postoperative hours is a sign of sepsis and an indication for an emergency laparoscopy.**

Classic signs of sepsis are worsening abdominal pain, fever, or leukocytosis. Obese patients tend to show these signs later than patients with normal BMI. Symptoms of staple line leakage also include dizziness and shortness of breath.

If an early leak is suspected perform relaparoscopy within the first 36 hours after surgery, locate the leak with the methylene blue test and oversew meticulously. In some cases placing a jejunal feeding tube can be advantageous.

Long persisting leaks should be repaired with a stent and local drainage. If a drainage is still in place relaparoscopy may not be necessary. Conservative treatment with stent placement or parenteral nutrition may be sufficient.

Adequate leakage management varies from case to case. Make sure to discuss the appropriate individual management with an experienced bariatric surgeon.

> **Early detection of a leak is essential to prevent the development of sepsis!**

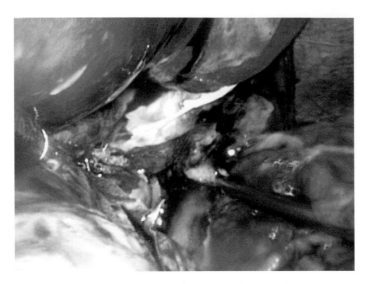

Positive methylene blue test with exudation of the dye caused by a leak.

c) Fistula

Fistula typically occurs as a late complication. It should be treated conservatively or gastroscopically by placing a stent.

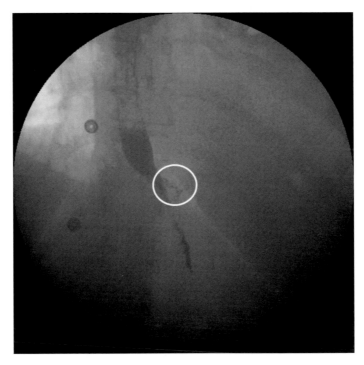

Postoperative development of a fistula.

d) Sleeve dilatation

Sleeve dilatation typically occurs as a late complication.

Reasons for this complication may be:
- the sleeve (i.e. antrum size) created during the operation is too large,
- the stomach is fixated due to posterior stomach wall adhesions that were not resected completely,
- the patient is eating too hastily,
- the patient is eating beyond a sensation of satiety, or
- the patient consumes carbonic acid-containing drinks.

Give a contrast agent under X-ray control or perform a multidetector computed tomography scan to confirm the diagnosis of a sleeve dilatation.

Evaluate a surgical revision. If possible perform a relaparoscopy.

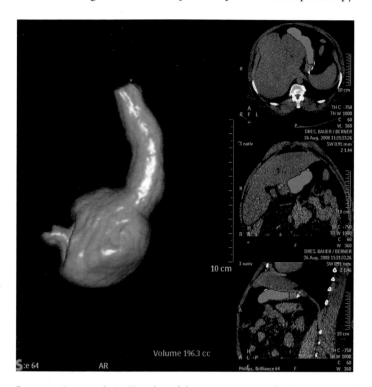

Postoperative prepyloric dilatation of the antrum 4 years after laparoscopic sleeve gastrectomy using a multidetector CT scanner.

e) Gastroesophageal reflux

Gastroesophageal reflux is a typical complication following sleeve gastrectomy. It often happens when a sleeve with a small volume (i.e. small antrum size) was created. If the gastroesophageal reflux persists, consider an RYGBP as a second-step procedure.

f) Sleeve necrosis

Sleeve necrosis is a very rare complication presumably caused by rupture or injury of the left gastric artery, which carries the main arterial blood supply for the stomach. Rehabilitation is achieved with an esophageal-jejunal anastomosis.

g) Functional stenosis due to torsion of the sleeve (kinking)

Functional stenosis typically occurs as a late postoperative complication. It is detected by upper GI-series or gastroscopy. If a functional stenosis is diagnosed perform a laparoscopic revision. Fixate the proximal sleeve to the diaphragm. If necessary remove the oversewing.

Bibliography

Adler R.I. & Terry B.E. (1977). Measurement and standardization of the gastric pouch in gastric bypass. *Surgery, Gynecology and Obstetrics*, 144: 762–763.

Agarwal S., Kini S.U. & Herron D.M. (2007). Laparoscopic sleeve gastrectomy for morbid obesity: a review. *Surgery for Obesity and Related Diseases*, 3: 189–194.

Aguilo Espases R., Lozano R., Navarro A.C., Regueiro F., Tejero E. & Salinas J.C. (2004). Gastrobronchial fistula and anastomotic esophagogastric stenosis after esophagectomy for esophageal carcinoma. *The Journal of Thoracic and Cardiovascular Surgery*, 127: 297–299.

Almogy G., Crookes P.F. & Anthone G.J. (2004). Longitudinal gastrectomy as a treatment for the high-risk super-obese patient. *Obesity Surgery*, 14: 492–497.

Arora S., Aggarwal R., Sevdalis N., Moran A., Sirimanna P., Kneebone R. & Darzi A. (2010). Development and validation of mental practice as a training strategy for laparoscopic surgery. *Surgical Endoscopy*, 24: 179–187.

Baltasar A., Bou R., Bengochea M., Serra C. & Cipagauta L. (2007). Use of a Roux limb to correct esophagogastric junction fistulas after sleeve gastrectomy. *Obesity Surgery*, 17: 1408–1410.

Baltasar A., Serra C., Pérez N., Bou R. & Bengochea M. (2006). Re-sleeve gastrectomy. *Obesity Surgery*, 16: 1535–1538.

Baltasar A., Serra C., Perez N., Bou R., Bengochea M. & Ferri L. (2005). Laparoscopic sleeve gastrectomy: a multi-purpose bariatric operation. *Obesity Surgery*, 15: 1124–1128.

Barboza E., Barboza A., Calmet F., Montes M., Ronceros V., Málaga G., Gotuzzo E., Sattui A., Portugal J., Mattos L., Bocanegra J., Vásquez F., Contardo M. & Arias Stella J. (2007). Life-saving total gastrectomy in abdominal sepsis after bariatric surgery of gastric sleeve. *Revista de Gastroenterología del Perú*, 27: 295–302.

Barzilai N., She L., Liu B.Q., Vuguin P., Cohen P., Wang J. & Rossetti L. (1999). Surgical removal of visceral fat reverses hepatic insulin resistance. *Diabetes*, 48: 94–98.

Behrus K.E., Smith C.D. & Sarr M.G. (1994). Prospective evaluation of gastric acid secretion and cobalamin absorption following gastric byapss for clinically severe obesity. *Digestive Diseases and Sciences*, 39: 315–320.

Bernante P., Foletto M., Busetto L., Pomerri F., Pesenti F.F., Pelizzo M.R. & Nitti D. (2006). Feasibility of laparoscopic sleeve gastrectomy as a revision procedure for prior laparoscopic gastric banding. *Obesity Surgery*, 16: 1327–1330.

Biertho L., Steffer R., Ricklin T.H., Horber F.F., Pomp A., Inabnet W.B., Herron D. & Gagner M. (2003). Laparoscopic gastric bypass versus laparoscopic adjustable gastric banding: a comparation study of 1200 cases. *Journal of the American College of Surgeons*, 197: 536–547.

Braghetto I., Korn O., Valladares H., Gutiérrez L., Csendes A., Debandi A., Castillo J., Rodríguez A., Burgos A.M. & Brunet L. (2007). Laparoscopic sleeve gastrectomy: surgical technique, indications and clinical results. *Obesity Surgery*, 17: 1442–1450.

Brega Massone P.P., Infante M., Valente M., Conti B., Carboni U. & Cataldo I. (2002). Gastrobronchial fistula repair followed by esophageal leak – rescue by transesophageal drainage of the pleural cavity. *The Journal of Thoracic and Cardiovascular Surgery*, 50: 113–116.

Brethauer S.A., Hammel J. & Schauer P.R. (2009). Systematic review of sleeve gastrectomy as a staging and primary bariatric operation. *Surgery for Obesity and Related Diseases*, 5: 469–475.

Buchwald H., Avidor Y., Braunwald E., Jensen M.D., Pories W., Fahrbach K. & Schoelles K. (2004). Bariatric surgery. A systematic review and meta-analysis. *Journal of the American Medical Association*, 292: 1724–1737.

Carmichael A.R. (1999). Treatment of morbid obesity. *Postgraduate Medical Journal*, 75: 7–12.

Carpenter W.B. (1874). *Principles of Mental Physiology: With their Applications to the Training and Discipline of the Mind and the Study of its Comorbid Conditions.* London: Henry S. King & Co.

Chazelet C., Verhaeghe P., Perterli R., Fennich S., Houdart R., Topart R., Tussiot J., Skawinski P., Seraille G., Catheline J.M., Merabet M., Dehaye B., Pautot V., Juglard G. & Sala J.J. (2009). La Sleeve gastrique isolée: résultats d'une serie multicentrique de 446 sleeve. *Journal de Chirurgie*, 146: 368–372.

Clinical Issues Committee of American Society for Metabolic and Bariatric Surgery. (2007). Sleeve gastrectomy as a bariatric procedure. *Surgery for Obesity and Related Diseases*, 3: 573–576.

Cohen R., Uzzan B., Bihan H., Khochtali I., Reach G. & Catheline J.M. (2005). Ghrelin levels and sleeve gastrectomy in super-super-obesity. *Obesity Surgery*, 15: 1024–1029.

Consten E.C., Gagner M., Pomp A. & Inabnet W.B. (2004). Decreased bleeding after laparoscopic sleeve gastrectomy with or without duodenal switch for morbid obesity using a stapled buttressed absorbable polymer membrane. *Obesity Surgery*, 14: 1360–1366.

Cottam D., Qureshi F.G., Mattar S.G., Sharma S., Holover S., Bonanomi G., Ramanathan & Schauer P. (2006). Laparoscopic sleeve gastrectomy as an initial weight-loss procedure for high-risk patients with morbid obesity. *Surgical Endoscopy*, 20: 859–863.

Crampton N.A., Izvornikov V. & Stubbs R.S. (1997). Silastic ring gastric bypass: results in 64 patients. *Obesity Surgery*, 7: 489–494.

Crampton N.A., Izvornikov V. & Stubbs R.S. (1997). Silastic ring gastric bypass: a comparison of two ring sizes: a preliminary report. *Obesity Surgery*, 7: 495–499.

Csendes A. & Burgos A.M. (2005). Size, volume and weight of the stomach in patients with morbid obesity compared to controls. *Obesity Surgery*, 15: 1133–1136.

Csendes A., Burdiles P., Díaz J.C., Maluenda F., Burgos A.M. & Recio M. (2002). Results of surgical treatment of morbid obesity. Analysis of 180 patients. *Revista médica de Chile*, 54: 3–9.

Csendes A., Burdiles P., Papapietro K., Díaz J.C., Maluenda F., Burgos A. & Rojas J. (2005). Results of gastric bypass plus resection of the distal excluded gastric segment in patients with morbid obesity. *Journal of Gastrointestinal Surgery,* 9: 121–131.

Dapri G., Vaz C., Cadiere G.B. & Himpens J. (2007). A prospective randomized study comparing two different techniques for laparoscopic sleeve gastrectomy. *Obesity Surgery,* 17: 1435–1441.

Daskalakis M., Berdan Y., Theodoridou S., Weigand G. & Weiner R.A. (2011). Impact of surgeon experience and buttress material on postoperative complications after laparoscopic sleeve gastrectomy. *Surgical Endoscopy,* 25: 88–97.

De Csepel J., Burpee S., Jossart G., Andrei V., Murakami Y., Benavides S. & Gagner M. (2001). Laparoscopic biliopancreatic diversion with a duodenal switch for morbid obesity: a feasibility study in pigs. *Journal of Laparoendoscopic & Advanced Surgical Techniques,* 11: 79–83.

Deitel M., Crosby R.D. & Gagner M. (2008). The First International Consensus Summit for Sleeve Gastrectomy (SG), New York City, October 25–27, 2007. *Obesity Surgery,* 18: 487–496.

Devbhandari M.P., Jain R., Galloway S. & Krysiak P. (2005). Benign gastro-bronchial fistula – an uncommon complication of esophagectomy: case report. *BMC Surgery,* 5: 16.

Elariny H., Gonzalez H. & Wang B. (2005). Tissue thickness of human stomach measured on excised gastric specimens of obese patients. *Surgical Technology International,* 14: 119–124.

Felberbauer F.X., Langer F., Shakeri-Manesch S., Schmaldienst E., Kees M., Kriwanek S., Prager M. & Prager G. (2008). Laparoscopic sleeve gastrectomy as an isolated bariatric procedure: intermediate-term results from a large series in three Austrian centers. *Obesity Surgery,* 18: 814–818.

Feltz D.L. & Landers D.M. (1983). The effects of mental practice on motor skill learning and performance: a meta-analysis. *Journal of Sport Psychology,* 5: 25–57.

Fobi M., Lee H., Igwe D., Felahy B., James E., Stanczyk M. & Fobi N. (2001). Band erosion: incidence, etiology, management and outcome after banded vertical gastric bypass. *Obesity Surgery,* 11: 699–707.

Fobi M.A.L., Lee H., Holmess R. & Cabinda D.G. (1998). Gastric bypass operation for obesity. *World Journal of Surgery,* 22: 925–935.

Frezza E.E. (2007). Laparoscopic vertical sleeve gastrectomy for morbid obesity. The future procedure of choice? Review. *Surgery Today,* 37: 275–281.

Frezza E.E., Reddy S., Gee L.L. & Wachtel M.S. (2009). Complications after sleeve gastrectomy for morbid obesity. *Obesity Surgery,* 19: 684–687.

Fuks D., Verhaeghe P., Brehant O., Sabbagh C., Dumont F., Riboulot M., Delcenserie R. & Regimbeau J.M. (2009). Results of laparoscopic sleeve gastrectomy: a prospective study in 135 patients with morbid obesity. *Surgery,* 145: 106–113.

Gagner M. & Rogula T. (2003). Laparoscopic reoperative sleeve gastrectomy for poor weight loss after biliopancreatic diversion with duodenal switch. *Obesity Surgery,* 13: 649–654.

Gagner M., Gumbs A.A., Milone L., Yung E., Goldenberg L. & Pomp A. (2008). Laparoscopic sleeve gastrectomy for the super-super-obese (body mass index >60 kg/m(2)). *Surgery Today,* 38: 399–403.

Gan S.S., Talbot M.L. & Jorgensen J.O. (2007). Efficacy of surgery in the management of obesity-related type 2 diabetes mellitus. *ANZ Journal of Surgery,* 77: 958-962.

Gehrer S., Kern B., Peters T., Christoffel-Courtin C. & Peterli R. (2010). Fewer nutrient deficiencies after laparoscopic sleeve gastrectomy (LSG) than after laparoscopic Roux-Y-gastric bypass (LRYGB)-a prospective study. *Obesity Surgery,* 20: 447–453.

Givon-Madhala O., Spector R., Wasserberg N., Beglaibter N., Lustigman H., Stein M., Arar N. & Rubin M. (2007). Technical aspects of laparoscopic sleeve gastrectomy in 25 morbidly obese patients. *Obesity Surgery,* 17: 722–727.

Güler A.K., Immenroth M., Berg T., Bürger T. & Gawad K.A. (2006). Evaluation einer neu konzipierten Operationsfibel durch den Vergleich mit einer klassischen chirurgischen Operationslehre. *Posterpräsentation auf dem 123. Kongress der Deutschen Gesellschaft für Chirurgie vom 02.-05. Mai 2006 in Berlin.*

Gumbs A.A., Gagner M., Dakin G. & Pomp A. (2007). Sleeve gastrectomy for morbid obesity. *Obesity Surgery,* 17: 962–969.

Hakeam H.A., O'Regan P.J., Salem A.M., Bamehriz F.Y. & Jomaa L.F. (2009). Inhibition of C-Reactive Protein in Morbidly Obese Patients After Laparoscopic Sleeve Gastrectomy. *Obesity Surgery,* 19: 456–460.

Hamoui N., Anthone G.J., Kaufman H.S. & Crookes P.F. (2006). Sleeve gastrectomy in the high-risk patient. *Obesity Surgery,* 16: 1445–1449.

Hansen E., Hajri T. & Abumrad N.N. (2006). Is all fat the same? The role of fat in the pathogenesis of the metabolic syndrome and type 2 diabetes mellitus. *Surgery,* 139: 711–716.

Hermreck A.S., Jewell W.R. & Hardin C.A. (1976). Gastric bypass for morbid obesity: results and complications. *Surgery,* 80: 498–505.

Hess D.S. & Hess D.W. (1998). Biliopancreatic diversion with a duodenal switch. *Obesity Surgery,* 8: 267–282.

Himpens J., Dapri D. & Cadière G.B. (2006). A prospective randomized study between laparoscopic gastric banding and laparoscopic isolated sleeve gastrectomy: results after 1 and 3 years. *Obesity Surgery,* 16: 1450–1456.

Holdstock C., Engstrom B.E., Ohrvall M., Lind L., Sundbom M. & Karlsson F.A. (2003). Ghrelin and adipose tissue regulatory peptides: effect of gastric bypass surgery in obese humans. *Journal of Clinical Endocrinology and Metabolism,* 88: 3177–3183.

Immenroth M. (2003). *Mentales Training in der Medizin. Anwendung in der Chirurgie und Zahnmedizin.* Hamburg: Kovac.

Immenroth M., Bürger T., Brenner J., Kemmler R., Nagelschmidt R., Eberspächer H. & Troidl H. (2005). Mentales Training in der Chirurgie. *Der Chirurg BDC,* 44: 21–25.

Immenroth M., Eberspächer H., Nagelschmidt M., Troidl H., Bürger T., Brenner J., Berg T., Müller M. & Kemmler R. (2005). Mentales Training in der Chirurgie – Sicherheit durch ein besseres Training. Design und erste Ergebnisse einer Studie. *MIC,* 14: 69–74.

Immenroth M., Bürger T., Brenner J., Nagelschmidt R., Eberspächer H. & Troidl H. (2007). Mental Training in surgical education: a randomized controlled trial. *Annals of Surgery,* 245: 385–391.

Immenroth M., Eberspächer H. & Hermann H.D. (2008). Training kognitiver Fertigkeiten. In J. Beckmann & M. Kellmann (Hrsg.), *Enzyklopädie der Psychologie (D, V, 2). Anwendungen der Sportpsychologie* (119–176). Göttingen: Hogrefe.

Juhan-Vague I. & Alessi M.C. (1997). PAI-1, obesity, insulin resistance and risk of cardiovascular events. *Journal of Thrombosis and Haemostasis,* 78: 656–660.

Karamanakos S.N., Vagenas K., Kalfarentzos F. & Alexandrides T.K. (2008). Weight loss, appetite suppression, and changes in fasting and postprandial ghrelin and peptide-YY levels after Roux-en-Y gastric bypass and sleeve gastrectomy: a prospective, double blind study. *Annals of Surgery,* 247: 401–407.

Karcz W.K., Kuesters S., Marjanovic G., Suesslin D., Kotter E., Thomusch O., Hopt U.T., Felmerer G., Langer M. & Baumann T. (2009). 3D-MSCT gastric pouch volumetry in bariatric surgery – preliminary clinical results. *Obesity Surgery,* 19: 508–516.

Karcz W.K., Marjanovic G., Grueneberger J., Baumann T., Bukhari W., Krawczykowski D. & Kuesters S. (2011). Banded sleeve gastrectomy using the GABP ring – surgical technique. *Obesity Facts,* 4: 77–80.

Karcz W.K., Suslin D., Baumann T., Utzolino S., Küsters S., Makarewicz W.J., Richter S., Tittelbach-Helmrich D., Höppner J., Thomusch O. & Marjanovic G. (2008). To have or not to have the ring: early and late surgical complications after banded Roux-en-Y gastric bypass. *Videosurgery (Wideochirurgia),* 3: 53–65.

Kasalicky M., Michalsky D., Housova J., Haluzik M., Housa D., Haluzikova D. & Fried M. (2008). Laparoscopic Sleeve Gastrectomy without an Over-Sewing of the Staple Line. *Obesity Surgery,* 18: 1257–1262.

Kellum J.M., De Maria E.J. & Sugerman H.J. (1998). The surgical treatment of morbid obesity. *Current Problems in Surgery,* 35: 791–878.

Lalor P.F., Tucker O.N., Szomstein S. & Rosenthal R.J. (2008). Complications after laparoscopic sleeve gastrectomy. *Surgery for Obesity and Related Diseases,* 4: 33–38.

Langer F.B., Bohdjalian A., Felberbauer F.X., Fleischmann E., Reza Hoda M.A., Ludvik B., Zacherl J., Jakesz R. & Prager G. (2006). Does gastric dilatation limit the success of sleeve gastrectomy as a sole operation for morbid obesity? *Obesity Surgery,* 16: 166–171.

Langer F.B., Reza Hoda M.A., Bohdjalian A., Felberbauer F.X., Zacherl J., Wenzl E., Schindler K., Luger A., Ludvik B. & Prager G. (2005) Sleeve gastrectomy and gastric banding: effects on plasma ghrelin levels. *Obesity Surgery*, 15: 1024–1029.

Lee C.M., Cirangle P.T. & Jossart G.H. (2007). Vertical gastrectomy for morbid obesity in 216 patients: report of two-year results. *Surgical Endoscopy*, 21: 1810–1816.

Lee J.H., Lee J.Y., Jang M.K., Lee J.Y., Kim K.H., Park J.Y., Lee J.H., Kim H.Y. & Yoo J.Y. (2005). Bronchogastric fistula. *Gastrointestinal Endoscopy*, 61: 289–290.

Lotze R.H. (1852). *Medicinische Psychologie und Physiologie der Seele*. Leipzig: *Weidmann'sche Buchhandlung*.

Mac Donald K.G. Jr., Long S.D., Swanson M.S., Brown B.M., Morris P., Dohm G.L. & Pories W.J. (1997). The gastric bypass operation reduces the progression and mortality of non-insulin-dependent diabetes mellitus. *Journal of Gastrointestinal Surgery*, 1: 213–220.

MacLean L.D., Rhode B.M., Sampalis J. & Forse R.A. (1993). Results of surgical treatment of obesity. *American Journal of Surgery*, 165: 155–162.

Marceau P., Biron S., Bourque R.A., Potvin M., Hould F.S. & Simard S. (1993). Biliopancreatic Diversion with a New Type of Gastrectomy. *Obesity Surgery*, 3: 29–35.

Marcuard S.P., Sinar D.R., Swanson M.S., Siberman J.F. & Levine J.S. (1989). Absence of luminal intrinsic factor after gastric bypass surgery for morbid obesity. *Digestive Diseases and Sciences*, 34: 1238–1242.

Mason E.E. & Ito C.H. (1969). Gastric bypass. *Annals of Surgery*, 170: 329–337.

Mason E.E. & Ito C.H. (1978). Graded gastric bypass. *World Journal of Surgery*, 2: 341–349.

McTernan C.L., McTernan P.G., Harte A.L., Levick P.L., Barnett A.H. & Kumar S. (2002). Resistin, central obesity, and type 2 diabetes. *The Lancet*, 359: 46–47.

Meir E. & Van Baden M. (1999) Adjustable silicone gastric banding and band erosion: personal experience and hypotheses. *Obesity Surgery*, 9: 191–193.

Melissas J., Koukouraki S., Askoxylakis J., Stathaki M., Daskalakis M., Perisinakis K. & Karkavitsas N. (2007). Sleeve gastrectomy: a restrictive procedure? *Obesity Surgery*, 17: 57–62.

Miller G.A. (1956). The magical number seven plus or minus two: some limits on our capacity for processing information. *Psychological Review*, 63: 81–97.

Milone L., Strong V. & Gagner M. (2005). Laparoscopic sleeve gastrectomy is superior to endoscopic intragastric balloon as a first stage procedure for super-obese patients (BMI > or =50). *Obesity Surgery*, 15: 612–617.

Mognol P., Chosidow D. & Marmuse J.P. (2005). Laparoscopic sleeve gastrectomy as an initial bariatric operation for high-risk patients: initial results in 10 patients. *Obesity Surgery*, 15: 1030–1033.

Mognol P., Chosidow D. & Marmuse J.P. (2006). Laparoscopic sleeve gastrectomy (LSG): review of a new bariatric procedure and initial results. *Surgical Technology International,* 15: 47–52.

Moon Han S., Kim W.W. & Oh J.H. (2005). Results of laparoscopic sleeve gastrectomy (LSG) at 1 year in morbidly obese Korean patients. *Obesity Surgery,* 15: 1469–1475.

Muccioli G., Tschop M., Papotti M., Deghenghi R., Heiman M. & Ghigo E. (2002). Neuroendocrine and peripheral activities of ghrelin: implications in metabolism and obesity. *European Journal of Pharmacology,* 440: 235–254.

Mui W.L., Ng E.K., Tsung B.Y., Lam C.C. & Yung M.Y. (2008). Laparoscopic Sleeve Gastrectomy in Ethnic Obese Chinese. *Obesity Surgery,* 18: 1571–1574.

Neto N.I., Godoy E.P., Campos J.M., Abrantes T., Quinino R., Barbosa A.L. & Fonseca C.A. (2007). Superior mesenteric artery syndrome after laparoscopic sleeve gastrectomy. *Obesity Surgery,* 17: 825–827.

Nguyen N.T., Longoria M., Gelfand D.V., Sabio A. & Wilson S.E. (2005). Staged laparoscopic Roux-en-Y: a novel two-stage bariatric operation as an alternative in the super-obese with massively enlarged liver. *Obesity Surgery,* 15: 1077–1081.

Niville E., Dams A. & Vlasselaers J. (2001). Lap-Band erosion: incidence and treatment. *Obesity Surgery,* 11: 744–747.

Nocca D., Krawczykowsky D., Bomans B., Noël P., Picot M.C., Blanc P.M., de Seguin de Hons C., Millat B., Gagner M., Monnier L. & Fabre J.M. (2008). A prospective multicenter study of 163 sleeve gastrectomies: results at 1 and 2 years. *Obesity Surgery,* 18: 560–565.

Ou Yang O., Loi K., Liew V., Talbot M. & Jorgensen J. (2008). Staged laparoscopic sleeve gastrectomy followed by Roux-en-Y gastric bypass for morbidly obese patients: a risk reduction strategy. *Obesity Surgery,* 18: 1575–1580.

Parikh M., Gagner M., Heacock L., Strain G., Dakin G. & Pomp A. (2008). Laparoscopic sleeve gastrectomy: does bougie size affect mean %EWL? Short-term outcomes. *Surgery for Obesity and Related Diseases,* 4: 528–533.

Peterli R., Steinert R.E., Wölnerhanssen B., Peters T., Christoffel-Courtin C., Borbély Y., Kern B., von Flüe M. & Beglinger C. (2012). Hormonal and Metabolic Implications of Weight loss after laparoscopic Roux-en-Y Gastric Bypass and Sleeve Gastrectomy: A Randomized, Prospective Trial. Submitted to *Obesity Surgery*.

Peterli R., Steinert R.E., Wölnerhanssen B., Peters T., Christoffel-Courtin C., Gass M., Kern B., von Flüe M. & Beglinger C. (2012). Metabolic and hormonal changes after laparoscopic Roux-en-Y gastric bypass and sleeve gastrectomy: A randomized, prospective trial. Submitted to *Obesity Surgery.*

Peterli R., Wölnerhanssen B., Peters T., Devaux N., Kern B., Christoffel-Courtin C., Drewe J., von Flüe M. & Beglinger C. (2009). Improvement in glucose metabolism after bariatric surgery: Comparison of laparoscopic Roux-en-Y gastric bypass and laparoscopic sleeve gastrectomy: a prospective randomized trial. *Annals of Surgery,* 250: 234–241.

Pramesh C.S., Sharma S., Saklani A.P. & Sanghvi B.V. (2001). Broncho-gastric fistula complicating transthoracic esophagectomy. *Diseases of the Esophagus,* 14: 271–273.

Quesada B.M., Roff H.E., Kohan G., Salvador Oria A. & Chiappetta Porras L.T. (2008). Laparoscopic sleeve gastrectomy as an alternative to gastric bypass in patients with multiple intraabdominal adhesions. *Obesity Surgery,* 18: 566–568.

Rabkin R.A., Rabkin J.M., Metcalf B., Lazo M., Rossi M. & Lehmanbecker L.B. (2003). Laparoscopic technique for performing duodenal switch with gastric reduction. *Obesity Surgery,* 13: 263–268.

Regan J.P., Inabnet W.B., Gagner M. & Pomp A. (2003). Early experience with two-stage laparoscopic Roux-en-Y gastric bypass as an alternative in the super-super obese patient. *Obesity Surgery,* 13: 861–864.

Roa P.E., Kaidar-Person O., Pinto D., Cho M., Szomstein S. & Rosenthal R.J. (2006). Laparoscopic sleeve gastrectomy as treatment for morbid obesity: technique and shortterm outcome. *Obesity Surgery,* 16: 1323–1326.

Rubin M., Yehoshua R.T., Stein M., Lederfein D., Fichman S., Bernstine H. & Eidelman L.A. (2008). Laparoscopic Sleeve Gastrectomy with Minimal Morbidity Early Results in 120 Morbidly Obese Patients. *Obesity Surgery,* 18: 1567–1570.

Sakamoto K., Ogawa M., Yamamoto S., Mugita N., Saishoji T., Azuma A.S. & Hayashida K. (1997). Closure of gastric tube-tracheal fistula by transposition of a pedicled sternocleidomastoid muscle flap. *Surgery Today,* 27: 181–185.

Santoro S. (2007). Technical Aspects in Sleeve Gastrectomy. *Obesity Surgery,* 17: 1534–1535.

Santoro S. (2008). Adaptive and Neuroendocrine Procedures: A New Pathway in Bariatric and Metabolic Surgery. *Obesity Surgery,* 18: 1343–1345.

Santoro S., Malzoni C.E., Velhote M.C.P., Milleo F.Q., Santo M.A., Klajner S., Damiani D. & Maksoud J.G. (2006). Digestive Adaptation with Intestinal Reserve: A neuroendocrine-based procedure for morbid obesity. *Obesity Surgery,* 16: 1371–1379.

Santoro S., Velhote M.C., Mechenas A.S.G., Malzoni C.E. & Strassmann V. (2003). Laparoscopic adaptive gastro-omentectomy as an early procedure to treat and prevent the progress of obesity. *Revista Brasileira de Videocirurgia,* 1: 96–102.

Santoro S., Velhote M.C.P., Malzoni C.E. Milleo F.Q., Klajner S. & Campos F.G. (2006). Preliminary results of digestive adaptation: a new surgical proposal to treat obesity based in physiology and evolution. *São Paulo Medical Journal,* 124: 192–197.

Schauer P.H.R., Ikramuddin S., Gourash W., Ramnanathan V. & Luketich J. (2000). Outcomes after laparoscopic Roux-en-Y gastric bypass for morbid obesity. *Annals of Surgery,* 232: 515–529.

Serra C., Baltasar A., Andreo L., Pérez N., Bou R., Bengochea M. & Chisbert J.J. (2007). Treatment of gastric leaks with coated self-expanding stents after sleeve gastrectomy. *Obesity Surgery,* 17: 866–872.

Serra C., Baltasar A., Pérez N., Bou R. & Bengochea M. (2006). Total gastrectomy for complications of the duodenal switch, with reversal. *Obesity Surgery,* 16: 1082–1086.

Shimomura I., Funahashi T., Takahashi M., Maeda K., Kotani K., Nakamura T., Yamashita S., Miura M., Fukuda Y., Takemura K., Tokunaga K. & Matsuzawa Y. (1996). Enhanced expression of PAI-1 in visceral fat: possible contributor to vascular disease in obesity. *Nature Medicine,* 2: 800–803.

Silecchia G., Boru C., Pecchia A., Rizzello M., Casella G., Leonetti F. & Basso N. (2006). Effectiveness of laparoscopic sleeve gastrectomy (first stage of biliopancreatic diversion with duodenal switch) on co-morbidities in super-obese high-risk patients. *Obesity Surgery,* 16: 1138–1144.

Skrekas G., Lapatsanis D., Stafyla V. & Papalambros A. (2008). One year after laparoscopic „tight" sleeve gastrectomy: technique and outcome. *Obesity Surgery,* 18: 810–813.

Smith C.D., Herks S.H.B., Behrus K.E., Fairbanky V.F., Kelly K.A. & Sarr M.G. (1993). Gastric acid secretion and vitamin B12 absoption after vertical Roux-en-Y gastric bypass for morbid obesity. *Annals of Surgery,* 218: 91–96.

Stroh C., Birk D., Flade-Kuthe R., Frenken M., Herbig B., Höhne S., Köhler H., Lange V., Ludwig K., Matkowitz R., Meyer G., Meyer F., Pick P., Horbach T., Krause S., Schäfer L., Schlensak M., Shang E., Sonnenberg T., Susewind M., Voigt H., Weiner R., Wolff S., Lippert H., Wolf A.M., Schmidt U. & Manger T. (Bariatric Surgery Working Group) (2009). A nationwide survey on bariatric surgery in Germany – Results 2005–2007. *Obesity Surgery,* 19: 105–112.

Stroh C., Birk D., Flade-Kuthe R., Frenken M., Herbig B., Höhne S., Köhler H., Lange V., Ludwig K., Matkowitz R., Meyer G., Pick P., Horbach T., Krause S., Schäfer L., Schlensak M., Shang E., Sonnenberg T., Susewind M., Voigt H., Weiner R., Wolff S., Wolf A.M., Schmidt U., Lippert H. & Manger T. (Bariatric Surgery Working Group) (2009). Results of Sleeve Gastrectomy-Data from a Nationwide Survey on Bariatric Surgery in Germany. *Obesity Surgery,* 19: 632–640.

Sugerman H.J., Kellum J.M., Engle K.M., Wolfe H., Starkey J.V., Birkenhauer R., Fletcher P. & Sawyer M.J. (1994). Gastric bypass for treating severe obesity. *The American Journal of Clinical Nutrition,* 55: 560–566.

Tagaya N., Kasama K., Kikkawa R., Kanahira E., Umezawa A., Oshiro T., Negishi Y., Kurokawa Y., Nakazato T. & Kubota K. (2009). Experience with Laparoscopic Sleeve Gastrectomy for Morbid Versus Super Morbid Obesity. *Obesity Surgery,* 19: 1371–1376.

Takata M.C., Campos G.M., Ciovica R., Rabl C., Rogers S.J., Cello J.P., Ascher N.L. & Posselt A.M. (2008). Laparoscopic bariatric surgery improves candidacy in morbidly obese patients awaiting transplantation. *Surgery for Obesity and Related Diseases,* 4: 159–164; discussion 164–165.

Tretbar L.L., Taylor T.L. & Sifers EC. (1976). Weight reduction. Gastric plication for morbid obesity. *Journal of the Kansas Medical Society,* 77: 488–490.

Thörne A., Lönnqvist F., Apelman J., Hellers G. & Arner P. (2002). A pilot study of long-term effects of a novel obesity treatment: omentectomy in connection with adjustable gastric banding. *International Journal of Obesity and Related Metabolic Disorders,* 26: 193–199.

Triantafyllidis G., Lazoura O., Sioka E., Tzovaras G., Antoniou A., Vassiou K. & Zacharoulis D. (2011). Anatomy and complications following laparoscopic sleeve gastrectomy: radiological evaluation and imaging pitfalls. *Obesity Surgery,* 21: 473–478.

Tucker O.N., Szomstein S. & Rosenthal R.J. (2008). Indications for sleeve gastrectomy as a primary procedure for weight loss in the morbidly obese. *Journal of Gastrointestinal Surgery,* 12: 662–667.

Uglioni B., Wolnerhanssen B., Peters T., Christoffel-Courtin C., Kern B. & Peterli R. (2009). Mid-term Results of Primary vs. Secondary Laparoscopic Sleeve Gastrectomy (LSG) as an Isolated Operation. *Obesity Surgery,* 19: 401–406.

Vidal J., Ibarzabal A., Romero F., Delgado S., Momblán D., Flores L. & Lacy A. (2008). Type 2 diabetes mellitus and the metabolic syndrome following sleeve gastrectomy in severely obese subjects. *Obesity Surgery,* 18: 1077–1082.

Weiner R.A., Theodoridou S. & Weiner S. (2011). Failure of laparoscopic sleeve gastrectomy: further procedure? *Obesity Facts,* 4 (suppl1): 42–46.

Weiner R.A., Weiner S., Pomhoff I., Jacobi C., Makarewicz W. & Weigand G. (2007). Laparoscopic sleeve gastrectomy – influence of sleeve size and resected gastric volume. *Obesity Surgery,* 17: 1297–1305.

Wilkinson L.H. & Peloso O.A. (1981). Gastric (Reservoir) Reduction for Morbid Obesity. *Archives of Surgery,* 116: 602–605.

Woelnerhanssen B., Peterli R., Steinert R.E., Peters T., Borbély Y. & Beglinger C. (2011). Effects of post-bariatric surgery weight loss on adipokines and metabolic parameters: Comparison of laparoscopic Roux-en-Y gastric bypass (LRYGB) and laparoscopic sleeve gastrectomy (LSG) – a prospective randomized trial. *Surgery for Obesity and Related Diseases*; 7: 561–568.

Yehoshua R.T., Eidelman L.A., Stein M., Fichman S., Mazor A., Chen J., Bernstine H., Singer P., Dickman R., Beglaibter N., Shikora S.A., Rosenthal R.J. & Rubin M. (2008). Laparoscopic sleeve gastrectomy – Volume and pressure assessment. *Obesity Surgery,* 18: 1083-1088.

Zundel N. & Hernandez J.D. (2010). Revisional surgery after restrictive procedures for morbid obesity. *Surgical Laparoscopy Endoscopy & Percutaneous Techniques,* 20: 338–343.

APPENDICES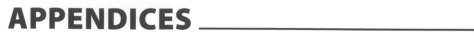

Marc Immenroth, PhD

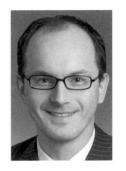

- Studied psychology (Diploma) and sports science (Master) in Heidelberg, Germany
- 1999–2006 Sports psychologist (including consultant to many top German athletes during their preparation for the World Championships and Olympics) and industrial psychologist (including consultant to Lufthansa Inc.)
- 2000 Research scientist at the University of Greifswald, Germany (Polyclinic for Restorative Dentistry and Periodontology)
- 2001–2004 Research scientist at the University of Heidelberg, Germany (Institute of Sports and Sports Science)
- 2002 Doctorate in psychology at the University of Heidelberg, Germany
- 2005–2006 Assistant lecturer at the University of Giessen, Germany (Institute of Sports)
- 2006–2008 Assistant professor at the University of Greifswald, Germany (Institute of Sports)
- 2006–2009 European Clinical Studies Manager at Ethicon Endo-Surgery (Europe) GmbH in Norderstedt, Germany
- 2009–2010 Marketing Manager and Sales Support at Ethicon Products, Johnson & Johnson MEDICAL GmbH in Norderstedt, Germany
- Since 2011 Senior Marketing Manager EP Germany & Plus Platform & Synthetic Absorbables D-A-CH, Johnson & Johnson MEDICAL GmbH in Norderstedt, Germany

Focus of Research and Work
- Mental training in sport, surgery and aviation
- Virtual reality in surgical education
- Coping with emotion and stress

Author of many scientific articles and textbooks on psychology, sports science and medicine

Jürgen Brenner, M.D.

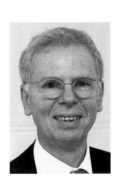

- Studied medicine in Hamburg, Germany
- 1972 Doctorate in medicine at the University of Hamburg, Germany
- 1972 Institute for Neuroanatomy, University of Hamburg, Germany
- 1974 Senior Resident at the Department of Surgery of the General Hospital Hamburg-Wandsbek, Germany
- 1981 Medical Director of the Department for Colorectal and Trauma Surgery at St. Adolf Stift Hospital in Reinbek, Germany
- 1987 Director for Surgical Research of Ethicon Inc. in Norderstedt, Germany
- 1989 Director of European Surgical Institute and Vice President Professional Education Europe of Ethicon Endo-Surgery (Europe) GmbH in Norderstedt, Germany
- 2004 Managing Director at Ethicon Endo-Surgery Germany in Norderstedt, Germany
- 2008–2011 Director of European Surgical Institute in Norderstedt, Germany
- Since 2011 Managing Director, Eric Krauthammer & Dr. Jürgen Brenner, Creative Team-Leadership

APPENDICES

Dr. Carl GmbH

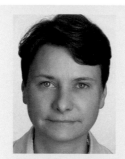

Indre Offermann, M.D.
Medical Writer

**European Surgical
Institute (ESI)**

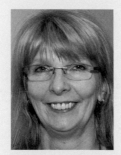

Maike Aukstinnis
Teamleader
Medical Training

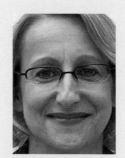

Astrid Künemund
Senior Manager
Medical Training

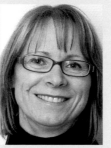

Annegret Röhling
Assistant ESI Director

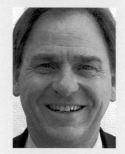

Detlev Ruge
Manager Event Technology

**Ethicon Endo-Surgery
Johnson & Johnson
MEDICAL GmbH**

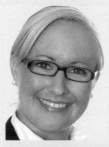

Ann-Katrin Güler, M.D.
Consultant Medical Products

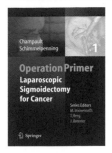
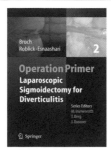
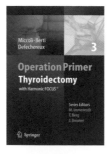
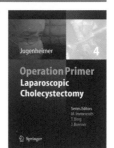
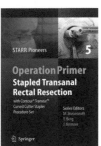
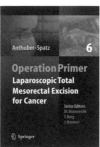
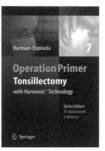
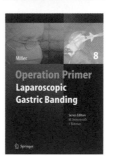
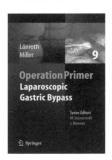
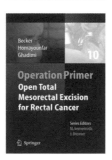
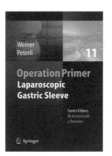
Volume 1: Laparoscopic Sigmoidectomy for Cancer   ISBN 978-3-540-78453-1

Volume 2: Laparoscopic Sigmoidectomy for Diverticulitis   ISBN 978-3-540-78451-7

Volume 3: Thyroidectomy with Harmonic FOCUS®   ISBN 978-3-540-85163-9

Volume 4: Laparoscopic Cholecystectomy   ISBN 978-3-540-92961-1

Volume 5: Stapled Transanal Rectal Resection with
Contour® Transtar™ Curved Cutter Stapler Procedure Set ISBN 978-3-540-92958-1

Volume 6: Laparoscopic Total Mesorectal Excision for Cancer   ISBN 978-3-642-04730-5

Volume 7: Tonsillectomy with Harmonic® Technology   ISBN 978-3-642-12747-2

Volume 8: Laparoscopic Gastric Banding   ISBN 978-3-642-19274-6

Volume 9: Laparoscopic Gastric Bypass   ISBN 978-3-642-23001-1

Volume 10: Open Total Mesorectal Excision (TME) for Rectal Cancer ISBN 978-3-642-23883-3

Volume 11: Laparoscopic Sleeve Gastrectomy   ISBN 978-3-642-23889-5

Titles in preparation

Video-assisted Thoracoscopic Lobectomy

Laparoscopic Hysterectomy

NOTES

NOTES